Edward G Ruppel

A Taste for Life

A Taste for Life

Recipes for a High-Protein Diet

Especially Suited for Hypoglycemia, Diabetes and Weight Reduction

Marcia Grad

Introduction by
R. Paul St. Amand, M.D.

Charles Scribner's Sons, New York

Library of Congress Cataloging in Publication Data

Grad, Marcia.
A taste for life.

Includes index.
1. High-protein diet. 2. Cookery for hypoglycemics.
3. Cookery for diabetics. 4. Reducing diets.
I. Title.
RM237.65.G7 641.5'638 75-22217
ISBN 0-684-14381-X

This book published simultaneously in the
United States of America and in Canada—
Copyright under the Berne Convention

1 3 5 7 9 11 13 15 17 19 v/c 20 18 16 14 12 10 8 6 4 2

Printed in the United States of America

ACKNOWLEDGMENTS

My deepest appreciation to Dr. R. Paul St. Amand for his keen interest and invaluable guidance. My gratitude to Constance Schrader for her inestimable assistance and support.

To my husband, Jerry, who patiently tasted my recipes, lost over thirty pounds on the Strict Diet and without whose creative ideas and constant encouragement this book would not have been completed.

To my children, Laura and Robert, who are bravely living low sugar lives in a children's world of cupcakes, candy and ice cream.

Contents

Foreword

Hypoglycemia (low blood sugar) is a poor name for this disease. Actually, low blood sugar, only part of the condition, occurs for about fifteen to thirty minutes several times a day. These cycles relate to carbohydrate intake. Other symptoms, such as fatigue, nervousness, irritability and depression, are present day and night regardless of blood sugar level.

Current studies are only beginning to uncover abnormalities in metabolism and endocrinology which might shed light on hypoglycemia. These abnormalities, rather than the transient fall in blood sugar, are the probable causes of the continuous symptoms.

Restricted carbohydrate intake, careful attention to diet and frequent meals have been found to correct all the symptoms of hypoglycemia in almost every patient. It is well to remember in any approach to the hypoglycemia syndrome that initially *NO* dietary lapse can be allowed or healing may not occur.

For the past several years, in treating patients with hypoglycemia, we have separated them into overweight and normal-weight categories. The overweight are given our version of a strict diet. Designed to deliver about thirty grams of carbohydrate, this diet allows the patient to eat as much as he requires to clear up symptoms of the disease and at the same time lose weight.

Normal-weight patients are given a liberal diet. They are permitted a wider range of food and of carbohydrates than those concerned also about their weight. Although the carbohydrate in an apple cannot be replaced by an equivalent amount of sugar or starch (flour), both forbidden foods, the Liberal Diet offers great freedom of choice. In hypoglycemia the quality of the carbohydrate is of prime importance; the quantity consumed of the tolerated ones is much less vital. Dietary indiscretions can have serious consequences.

Those who would follow either the Strict Diet or the Liberal Diet included in this book should do so with the agreement of their physician. Only their doctor is familiar with the necessary details of their condition. He may have sound medical reasons for restricting certain items included in these diets. His guidance is essential to your final success.

R. Paul St. Amand, M.D.

Introduction

This recipe collection began with my own need to remain faithful to a high-protein diet for an extended period of time. For more than one year after being diagnosed hypoglycemic, I followed a diet regime consisting mainly of broiled fish, hamburgers and scrambled eggs. Eating six such meals per day—as required—became difficult to the point of desperation.

I then decided something had to be done about my self-inflicted force-feedings. As a first step, I wrote a letter to the hospital where I had been treated, requesting recipes and recipe sources for a hypoglycemic diet. The hospital dietician was not very helpful. Then I questioned my physician and many people I know who have low blood sugar and came up with a few basic ideas. Finally, I began to haunt bookstores and the library. During this search for recipes, I came across information about the diet.

When my husband went to his physician for a physical examination and was told that his cholesterol and triglyceride levels were dangerously elevated, I was preparing my meals separately from his and our children's. The doctor put him on the same diet as mine, saying that eliminating sugar and reducing starch would lower those levels. I was extremely concerned about his eating eggs every morning and butter, cheeses and beef—most of the foods not allowed on the customary low-fat, low-cholesterol diet.

I began to read every piece of new research literature available and became overwhelmingly convinced that this low-carbohydrate approach was, by far, the one most likely to succeed. Evidence of success came early when, after only one month on the diet, my husband's blood tests revealed a 50 percent decrease in his triglyceride level and a 30 percent decrease in serum cholesterol. In addition, by the end of the second month he had lost over thirty pounds!

In affluent countries, at least one out of every three males over forty-five years of age dies of heart disease.[1] I believe that my husband's chances of becoming one of those afflicted have been greatly reduced by his adherence to the diet. The evidence is extremely convincing that the overconsumption of sugar is deeply implicated in the current epidemics of what Dr. John Yudkin has called the "malnutrition of affluence" [2]—heart disease, diabetes (one in every five Americans will have it or its inherited trait by 1980 [3]), overweight and obesity (three million adolescents and nearly 40 percent of the adult population of this country [4]), dental caries and ulcers. Hypoglycemia is conservatively estimated to affect ten million Americans. Many surveys have placed the number far above that estimate.

The Department of Agriculture tells us that one hundred million people, or approximately half the population, are not getting a good diet.[5] Substitution of refined, unnatural carbohydrates for the natural, unrefined ones has been widely blamed for a whole group of medical conditions. The loss of fiber resulting from this substitution has been said to cause varicose veins, diverticular disease, cancer of the colon, hemorrhoids and constipation.[6]

Once I realized that sugar and refined carbohydrates are the main items our diet eliminates, it occurred to me that I was not only creating horrendous problems and dreaded inconvenience with my dual dietary approach (separate meals for the children), but that I was doing the children a disservice by going out of my way to prepare foods for them that were nutritionally inferior to those we were eating and, in addition, were potentially harmful to their health.

Because the trait that predisposes one to metabolize carbohydrates improperly is inherited, and the typical American high-carbohydrate diet (50 percent of those carbohydrates being consumed in the form of sugar) may encourage the development of this trait, eventually blooming into hypoglycemia, diabetes and/or coronary heart disease, it became shockingly obvious that I had to question seriously the amounts of sugar and kinds of carbohydrate foods my children were consuming.

My husband and I have shown ourselves to be carbohydrate-intolerant but, at present, there is no way to determine whether our children have inherited this trait—though nutritionists at the Carbohydrates Nutrition Laboratory in collaboration with scientists in Israel are currently developing such a test.[7] The only safe approach, then, is to limit strictly their intake of the one thing that can make this trait become a serious illness. That one thing is sugar. If you have a family history of overweight, obesity, hypoglycemia or diabetes and you continue to allow yourself and your children to eat our average Western diet, there is strong evidence that you are taking a serious gamble with your health and theirs!

In April 1972, there was an international scientific convention in Oberusel near Frankfurt, West Germany. Thirty-five of the world's greatest experts on obesity, diabetes, arteriosclerosis and metabolism attended by personal invitation. After three days of discussing the relationship of diabetes and vascular disease, they voted unanimously to recommend the urgent limitation of human ingestion of sugar.[8]

Scientific conventions in Norway, Italy and the United States have supported the opinion of the West German convention.[9] In April 1973 our own Select Committee on Nutrition and Human Needs held three days of hearings on sugar. World-recognized researchers in the fields of nutrition, metabolism, diabetes and heart disease who appeared before the committee called for drastic reductions in sugar consumption. Especially emphasized was the urgency of putting strict limitations on the amounts consumed by children from birth, since the noxious effect is said to be cumulative and may take years to become apparent.[10] It is believed that damage to the arteries and metabolic changes characteristic of diabetes begin in early childhood and have a long incubation period.[11] Testimony was given that people born with a tendency toward diabetes can prevent the disease and all of its complications (blindness—diabetes is the leading cause in the country;[12] heart disease—causes thirty-five thousand diabetic deaths annually;[13] kidney damage, etc.), by a strict limitation of dietary sugar from birth.[14] It was strongly recommended that there be a comprehensive official government study conducted to determine exactly how much reduction is necessary.

So I did my own children a tremendous favor, one they will continuously thank me for with their good health: I finally began to prepare their foods as I did ours. The hypoglycemic diet became a family affair.

Experimenting with allowed foods, slowly, over a period of more than three years, I produced this collection. It includes adaptations of my favorite prehypoglycemia recipes and new recipes that came out of my long sieges in the kitchen. The kitchen, incidentally, is not my favorite place. Because others, like me, cannot or choose not to spend hours following involved "scratch" recipes, most recipes included here can be made quickly and prepared ahead of time.

More than half the known hypoglycemics are overweight.[15] Therefore, the diet recommended here was formulated to treat those who are both hypoglycemic and overweight. Also, these recipes can be easily adapted to many currently popular weight-reduction diets and to various other restricted medical diets as well.

High-protein, low-carbohydrate, moderate-fat diets are increasingly recommended for a variety of medical problems. They have proven to provide more effective control over diabetes than the conventional "everything included" diets, to be more successful with ulcer patients than the old gastric or bland diet (sugar is a stomach irritant[16]), to be more effective for long-term weight control than the "general caloric reduction" diets[17] and they are often advised for alcoholics, certain drug addicts and schizophrenics.

I prepare only recipes from this book in my home. My husband is now thin and feels well, our children eat more healthful meals and substitute nutritious desserts for most of their sweets.

Company enjoys the same dietary benefits from eating in our home as we do and I would not consider serving them what I now know to be substandard food. I consider any meal prepared without sugar a special gift to those who consume it. The meals are appetizing, delicious and can only contribute to their well-being.

We are vocal about our views on sugar and they are not only respected by friends and relatives, but have been fully accepted by many of them as partly evidenced by the fact that they have requested recipes for use in their own homes.

Uninteresting, repetitious meals and snacks are likely to lead to diet cheating. Accept the diet as your unalterable way of life. If you allow these recipes to help you prepare food that is aesthetically pleasing and physically satisfying, you will be richly rewarded with the satisfaction of knowing you are making a significant contribution to your own and your family's good health.

NOTES

1. John Yudkin, M.D., *Sweet and Dangerous* (New York: Peter H. Wyden, Inc., 1972), p. 83.
2. John Yudkin, M.D., "Dietary Sugar and Disease," in *Sugar in Diet, Diabetes and Heart Diseases,* Hearings before the Senate Select Committee on Nutrition and Human Needs of the United States Senate, Series 73/ND2 (Washington: Government Printing Office, 1973), p. 233.
3. *Sugar in Diet, Diabetes and Heart Diseases, op. cit.,* p. 146.
4. *Ibid.*
5. *Ibid.*
6. *Ibid.,* p. 242.
7. *Ibid.,* p. 149.
8. *Ibid.,* p. 217.
9. "Sugar Harmful? Scientist Says Yes," Special to the *Gainesville* (Fla.) *Sun,* February 13, 1973, in *Sugar in Diet, Diabetes and Heart Diseases, op. cit.,* p. 199.
10. A. M. Cohen, M.D., "High Sucrose Intake As a Factor in the Development of Diabetes and Its Vascular Complications," in *Sugar in Diet, Diabetes and Heart Diseases, op. cit.,* p. 192.
11. *Sugar in Diet, Diabetes and Heart Diseases, op. cit.,* p. 237.
12. "How Sweet It's Not," CBS telecast on diabetes, March 24, 1975.
13. *Sugar in Diet, Diabetes and Heart Diseases, op. cit.,* p. 146.
14. *Ibid.,* p. 164.
15. NBC News documentary on hypoglycemia, January 1973.
16. Yudkin, "Dietary Sugar and Disease," *op. cit.,* p. 236.
17. Yudkin, *Sweet and Dangerous, op. cit.,* pp. 56–57.

Part One

Notes from the Author

On Children

Do you think that in order to "un-sugar" your children's diet and rid it of the highly refined foods about which we have been warned, that you must:

turn them into miniature "nutrition nuts"?

inflict upon them unfair, in some cases nearly impossible dietary restrictions?

make emotional or sociological misfits of them by changing their eating habits too drastically?

make them resent you for forcing them to be different from their friends?

deprive them of all the foods they most desire?

I admit to having had these doubts and many others as well when I first began working toward a better diet for my own two children. Fortunately for us and for you, who want to do the same for your children, none of these doubts were ever realized. Things went along very smoothly, for the most part, as the children learned to apply new dietary knowledge to their own eating habits.

It means a great deal to me that both Laura, age nine, and Robert, age six, be well-adjusted and happy as well as in good physical health. Although I would be very pleased if they never again consumed any sugar, I think that this is an unrealistic approach because of the dietary world in which they must grow up. I believe that I have found a way to compromise with their childhood desires without compromising their health.

I have taught them to go on the premise that sugar and large quantities of "junk" (a term they use for all highly processed foods) may be harmful to them. Instead of thinking that they are being deprived of wonderful things, they often express concern for the well-being of friends who habitually eat too many junk foods. Both Laura and Robbie often relate humorous stories, usually over dinner, of experiences they have had while observing other children eating lunch at school or while attempting to explain their own eating habits to friends.

Because school cafeteria food is notoriously high in starch and sugar and, in addition, is often poorly prepared, my children eat only an occasional lunch there. If the dessert served that day is not their favorite, they do not eat it, preferring to have something they would really appreciate at another time. Because they infrequently eat sweets, they are particular about them. They pick and choose foods with amazing ability in order not to "waste a dessert" on something about which they are not extremely enthusiastic.

I am frequently asked what my children tote to school for lunch. I pack either meat left over from a previous night's dinner, cheese, an egg or seafood salad. Sometimes I put the food into a little container; other times I use it as filling in a Stretch-Cut Gluten Bread sandwich (p. 143). I mix green and yellow fresh vegetable sticks, half a piece of fruit or a container of water-packed, canned fruit and send packets of nuts or sugar-free, whole-grain crackers with them. I do occasionally pack a peanut butter and jelly sandwich but neither the filling nor the bread contains any sugar and I do not rely on the sandwich to provide the entire protein portion of the lunch. A few potato chips—once in a while—the brand which contains only potatoes, salt and oil, add variety. The children regard their potato chips as a harmless non-food—a dessert of sorts to be eaten only with a complete, nutritious meal. I avoid barbecue snack products because they contain dextrose in addition to a generous helping of other chemicals. They purchase white milk from the school.

After-school snacks include such things as milk with

tuna or cheese, sometimes peanut butter on crackers, cream cheese on gluten toast with Cinnamon Sprinkle (p. 115) or fruit with or without cottage cheese. I have tried to teach Laura and Robbie to select the kinds of snacks which will help keep their blood sugar levels fairly even. Although I often have sugarless desserts prepared which are as nutritious as many entrees, I encourage the children to reserve them for after dinner. I consider it a serious mistake to allow children to develop the habit of eating any dessert after every meal and, certainly, between meals when they are known to be the most damaging. It would be all too easy later in their lives for them to continue eating desserts frequently though they may no longer be the wholesome ones they now eat.

At this point I would like to put your mind at ease about using sugar substitutes in your children's foods. I made a real project of researching this matter. I am thoroughly convinced that sugar substitutes are totally harmless and that sugar is so dangerously harmful that the choice of one over the other seems automatic. Dr. George D. Campbell of South Africa has found these substitutes to be "totally free of significant toxic effects in humans." Dr. John Yudkin and his family use exclusively artificial sweeteners in their own home. The work of many other scientists supports their conclusions.

At school and birthday parties where nut cups are filled with candy and juice cups with punch (a phenomenon I cannot understand) and a larger selection of sweets are served in one sitting than either of my children receive in three weeks, Laura chooses one or two things she likes best and either gives the rest away or brings it home to eat at another time. Robbie is very proud of himself when he has exercised restraint in this regard. Because this exercise in self-control brings out positive feelings in the children, I do not think it too much to expect of even a six-year-old that he eat such foods only on special occasions, and even then in moderation.

Because our home contains neither sugar nor products containing it and because I cook totally sugar-free, the only time my children consume any is when they are away from home. As long as they keep exercising what I proudly consider their uncanny good judgment, even in my absence, their total intake will continue to follow the recommendations of those scientists who fear for the health of all our children.

Athough at times it may seem that dietary changes are a real challenge—even children's chewable vitamins contain sugar—the most difficult obstacles can be overcome. I once considered Halloween such an obstacle. We have developed a system which has interested many people who have been attempting to reduce their children's sugar intake.

Both children go trick-or-treating with their friends, collecting candy from all over the neighborhood. When they return home, they count, sort and negotiate exchanges with each other. Unwrapped candy is discarded; each child then chooses a few favorites, eats one and puts what remains in our cupboard to be doled out as occasional dinner desserts. We put all the rest of the candy in the freezer. After several weeks when their friends' reserves are running low, Laura and Robbie conduct their annual candy sale. It is always a huge success and the proceeds are used to buy themselves toys.

A whole new reward system has been set up in our family. We often reward the children by taking them somewhere they want very much to go or by buying them a toy they may want. They are not ever given food as a prize for any reason.

You can change the course of your children's lives. When the United States government does its full-scale investigation on sugar and finally makes formal recommendations for the drastic reduction of sugar which many scientists think will inevitably follow, you and your family will not be among those who have already consumed hundreds of times the recommended amount. You will not have caused needless exposure of your family to the most frightening, least understood, most rampant diseases of the century!

On Food Shopping

Get into the habit of reading labels! An unbelievable amount of sugar is indiscriminately added to most of your foods without your consent and usually without your knowledge. There is sugar in most bottled, canned and packaged foods.

The picture is still an encouraging one, however, for items such as sugarless orange and tomato juices, salad dressings, tomato paste, sauce and whole canned tomatoes are readily available. Sugarless frozen vegetables and fruits, major brands of canned chicken and beef broth, even hot dogs are in the regular food sections of most supermarkets. Our favorite gluten bread, the brand with which I have achieved the best results with recipes appearing in this book, can also be easily found. (Sometimes it is kept in the frozen food section because it contains no preservatives.) None of these products are labeled dietetic.

Though most companies may add sugar to a particular product, there is usually at least one who makes that same item without the sugar. Thoroughly examine all labels and compare ingredients in different brands of similar products. You may already be using some of these sugarless foods without having been aware of what an excellent choice of brands you have made.

Though the same price, availability, flavor and convenience apply to both sugared and sugarless tomato sauce, for example, pathetically millions of shoppers unknowingly choose the former, unnecessarily raising their sugar intake.

A high-protein diet does not have to be expensive. Some products, frozen fruits for instance, cost less when they have not had sugar added. The less expensive cuts of meat are at least as nutritious as the cuts costing considerably more. Eggs are a fabulous protein buy and can be turned into scrumptious dinner entrees. For Liberal dieters, wheat germ can help supply critical protein and other essential nutrients at a very low cost. Once I outgrew its stigma, I found wheat germ to be useful in a variety of ways. I cook with it by adding some to recipes calling for Gluten Bread Crumbs. Since ¼ cup of wheat germ contains 9 grams of protein and 13 grams of high-quality carbohydrate, I often use it to enhance the nutritional value of my children's occasional bowl of sugarless cereal. Powdered non-fat milk is also a versatile, inexpensive supplier of protein.

When figuring the cost of the diet, money saved on junk foods and the money which will probably be saved on medical and dental bills must be considered. My own dietary indiscretions have already cost me much in addition to money. There is no way to buy back good health at any price once it has been destroyed!

Your shopping success is practically guaranteed if you have:

a KNOWLEDGE of the dangers of continuing what may be disastrous shopping patterns, an AWARENESS of what products actually contain and how their contents affect you,

a DESIRE to change those habit patterns which are undesirable, and

a WILLINGNESS to learn a new approach to food shopping.

Purchase cheeses which are, perhaps, new to you. Use them in place of the standard ones that may have become tiresome. Shop for a variety of allowed foods to give variety to your diet. Regularly buy both light and heavy cream, sour cream (delicious with fresh strawberries), plenty of eggs, sugarless canned diet fruits (as allowed) and avocados. Have nuts handy for those potentially dangerous snack urges. Keep a stock of unflavored gelatin, flavored diet gelatins and, if allowed, puddings.

Salad vegetables should be chosen with some imagination. Many kinds of leaf lettuce are more nutritious and less expensive than head lettuce. These also lend a welcome change in flavor and texture to salads.

Store canned tuna and salmon to have as snacks and "emergency" meals. For coffee drinkers, decaffeinated coffee is a must. Purchase sugarless diet sodas and a good sugar substitute. Remember, good nutrition and interesting diet cooking start in the food market.

On Time Savers

A blender and hermetic-seal bag appliance, relatively inexpensive items, are invaluable aids to diet cooking. The blender prepares many of the basic recipes most efficiently. Hermetically sealed bags allow sauces and various hard-to-keep foods to be refrigerated for long periods of time. Foods may be frozen and then reheated in the bags with a minimum of effort and no cleaning up.

Prepare double recipes whenever possible and freeze half for a future high-protein meal or meals. Leftovers often solve the snack problem, too. By preparing a little extra you save yourself time and work later on.

For convenience, it is wise to prepare and store a supply of basic ingredients for the recipes. Cooking is so much easier when such items as Gluten Bread Crumbs or Basic Tomato Sauce are ready for use. Chopped nuts can be refrigerated in a sealed jar. Batches of chicken and beef broth can be poured into ice cube trays and frozen. (One tray hold approximately two cups of broth.) The broth cubes, kept in plastic bags, are great for quick soups, sauces and gravies.

You'll soon develop your own techniques to save time, effort and money—techniques that will work well with your life style and good nutrition.

On Spices and Extracts

Make it an adventure to buy one new spice or extract each week. Experiment with the new taste; try adding the new spice to a familiar old dish or to a new one. Note the flavors which you and your family enjoy most. Spices are important to creative cooking and creative cooking is what helps to keep you on the diet.

Living without pineapple, oranges, cherries and some other fruits is far easier when the desire for their flavor is satisfied. The "banana urge" is fairly easy to avoid if you have just eaten a large portion of custard made with flavorful banana extract.

Some brands of imitation rum, brandy and coconut contain a small amount of sugar that is well tolerated by most hypoglycemics; however, it is preferable to use one of the sugarless brands available at many food markets and health food stores.

Purse, Pocket or Automobile

Life is easiest when you are well prepared to remain on your diet outside your home and traveling. It is very helpful to have the following items with you at all times:

Small packages of sugar substitute

Small packages of instant decaffeinated coffee

Gram counter

A copy of your diet, unless you are thoroughly familiar with it

A small bag of allowed nuts

A small packet, jar or container of ketchup and salad dressing

Many sugarless products are now available in packages that can be conveniently carried in pocket or purse.

A Word about Snacks

When you know you will be out at snack time, prepare for it by taking small packets of food with you. Cheese slices, beef jerky, a slice of cold meat or a stuffed egg all travel well. Other suggestions:

Tuna, salmon or chicken salad and a plastic fork (or chopsticks)

Cold meats or leftovers in a plastic bag

Consider where you are going and where you will be when you want to eat the food. Selecting the right food is important; never skip a meal or snack that is scheduled on your diet.

In ordering a snack at a restaurant, à la carte orders of meat or fish are usually the best choices. The appetizer sections of menus often list small servings of foods that would be suitable. Seafood salads are good when there is enough of the seafood to provide the necessary protein. Eating anything listed on the diet is probably better than skipping the snack entirely.

Restaurants

Many restaurant menus boldly state, "No Substitutions." Yet, I have found that nearly every eating establishment, from the highest quality one to the neighborhood hamburger stand, will courteously bend the rules a little when they know a customer is on a restricted medical diet. A good waiter or waitress can usually find a sympathetic chef who will prepare tuna salad without the customary sweet pickle relish or serve lobster tails with tomato slices rather than potato.

Do not hesitate to inquire about the ingredients of a particular dish. Does it contain sugar or flour? Most chefs will gladly supply the necessary information. Also, do not be timid. For instance, send that gluten bread you brought with you to the chef and ask that it be substituted for the rice or noodles usually served with a dish. More often then not, he will oblige without further ado. Remember, it is far easier, both physically and emotionally, to ask such a thing than to scrape and pick at your meal in an attempt to avoid foods not allowed on the diet. The less you tempt yourself the easier it is to exert full control.

Isn't it better to ask that a particular food be left off your plate than to have it served and try meekly to refrain from "just tasting it"? Dieting is difficult enough without making it more so by eating a complete meal staring at a forbidden, but desirable food. A "taste" only whets your appetite for more. One bite of forbidden food can nullify a week of dieting and will, most likely, put weight on you. A lapse from your diet when you are battling hypoglycemia or some other medical problem means chancing symptom aggravation or reappearance.

The usual "diet plates" offered by many restaurants are not necessarily on your diet. Most often they consist of, among other things, fruit canned in sugar-laden syrup. If you order such a dish, be sure to request fresh, unsweetened strawberries or cantaloupe in place of such fruit.

On nights when you have an eight o'clock dinner reservation, remember to eat a snack between five and six o'clock. Then, if you are not served until nine, you have not gone five or six hours without food. It is no treat to eat that meal out if you feel ill. A hypoglycemic who skips that dinner hour snack can practically count on not enjoying his late dinner!

Personal experience has taught me that attempting to eat in restaurants featuring only foreign foods is difficult unless you are familiar with what the foods are and how they are prepared. If your chosen eating spot is new to you, call ahead to find out what they serve that you are allowed to eat.

When in doubt, it is wiser to order plain foods and know that you are remaining true to your diet. Remember, you still can enjoy the treat of having someone else prepare and serve the meal to you.

Bleu cheese, Roquefort and oil and vinegar dressings are sometimes safe to order; to be sure, ask what they contain. If you are a 1000 Island or Russian dressing lover, beware of the sugar and sweet pickle in them. "Emergency 1000 Island Dressing" solves the problem. Ask for mayonnaise on the side and a lemon wedge. Combine salt, pepper and the package of diet ketchup you carry with you. Spoon it over the salad. The dressing is quite tasty.

Strict Diet for Hypoglycemia and Weight Reduction

Choose food from the following list.

MEATS AND FISH

All meats (including sugarless cold cuts)
All fowl and game
All fish and shellfish

Note: Most cold cuts are cured with sugar. Check labels for exceptions.

DAIRY PRODUCTS

Eggs, any style
All natural cheeses (including bleu, cheddar, cream, gouda, Swiss, etc., cottage and ricotta—½ cup limit)
American cheese (1 slice per day limit)
Cream (sweet, sour)
Butter and margarine

FRUITS

Fresh coconut
Avocado (½ per day limit) *or*
Cantaloupe (¼ per day limit) *or*
Strawberries (6–8 per day limit)
and
Lemon juice (2 Tbsp. per day limit) *or*
Lime juice (2 Tbsp. per day limit)

NUTS

(12 per day limit)

Almond	Hazel	Pistachio
Brazil	Hickory	Sunflower seeds (small handful)
Butternut	Macadamia	
Filbert	Pecan	Walnut

VEGETABLES

Asparagus
Bean sprouts
Broccoli
Brussels sprouts
Cabbage (1 cup limit)
Cauliflower
Celery
Cervelat
Chard
Chicory
Chinese cabbage (2 cup limit)
Chives
Cucumber
Eggplant
Endives
Escarole
Greens (mustard, beet)
Kale
Leeks
Lettuce (any type)
Mushrooms
Okra
Olives
Parsley
Peppers (green, red)
Pickles (dill, sour—limit 1)
Pimiento
Radish
Rhubarb
Salad greens
Sauerkraut
Spinach
Squash (summer, yellow, zucchini)
String beans
Tomatoes
Water chestnuts
Watercress

DESSERTS

Use only products made with artificial sweeteners.
Sugarless, diet gelatins
Sugarless custard with cream
Sugarless cheese cake without crust

DRINKS

Club soda
Sugarless diet sodas and sugarless quinine water (but no cola)
Decaffeinated coffee
Weak tea only (or herb tea)
Bourbon, cognac, gin, rum, scotch, vodka, dry wine

Note: One alcoholic beverage per day can be tolerated by most hypoglycemics after 1 month on the diet. Use discretion as individual tolerance levels vary.

CONDIMENTS AND SPICES

All spices (including seeds)
All imitation flavorings
Horseradish
Sauces such as hollandaise, mayonnaise, mustard, soy, tartar, Worcestershire, ketchup (sugarless only)

MISCELLANEOUS

Oil (all types) and fats
Caviar
Sugarless salad dressings
Vinegar

Liberal Diet for Hypoglycemia and Weight Maintenance

Add the following food to the Strict Diet listing.

FRUITS

Apples
Apricots
Blackberries (½ cup limit)
Blueberries (½ cup limit)
Boysenberries
Casaba melon (1 wedge limit)
Grapefruit
Grapefruit juice (unsweetened)
Honeydew melon (1 wedge limit)
Lemons
Limes
Nectarines
Plums
Oranges
Orange juice (unsweetened)
Papaya (½ melon limit)
Peaches
Pears
Raspberries (½ cup limit)
Strawberries
Tangerines
Tomato juice

VEGETABLES

Artichokes
Beets
Carrots
Onions
Peas
Pumpkin
Squash, winter
Turnip

MILK

Whole
Low-fat
Non-fat
Buttermilk
Powdered milk
Plain yogurt (avoid brands which contain starch or sugar)

NUTS

Cashews
Peanuts
Soya nuts

BREADS

One slice three times per day of white (least desirable), whole wheat, protein or light rye.

Best to use gluten or soya—no more than 2 slices at any one time

DESSERTS

Sugarless diet puddings (½ cup serving per day limit)

MISCELLANEOUS

Carob powder
Flour—gluten or soya only
Gravy—made with gluten or soya flour only
Wheat germ—used to fortify foods
2 tacos *or* 2 enchiladas

Each hypoglycemic's tolerance for listed foods will vary. Judge your tolerance level by how you feel and adjust your intake of foods accordingly.

Foods to Avoid Strictly

Sweet wines, fruit brandy and champagne
All soft drinks except those listed
Baked beans
Blackeyed peas (Cowpeas)
Lima beans
Potatoes
Corn
Popcorn
Bananas
Dried fruits
Barley
Rice
Pastas (spaghettis—all types)
Burritos
Tamales
Sweets of any kind

Do not use products which contain dextrose, glucose, hexitol, maltose, sucrose, honey, caffeine or starch.

Substitutions for Adapting Non-diet Recipes
Changes to Adapt Ingredients for Strict Diet

When recipe calls for:	*Substitute:*
Sugar	Sugar substitute or vanilla extract
1 Tbsp. cornstarch	Unflavored gelatin or 2 Tbsp. gluten flour
Whole milk	1 part light cream to 1 part water
Low- or non-fat milk	1 part light cream to 5 parts water
1 cup buttermilk	½ cup light cream, ½ cup water and 1 Tbsp. vinegar or lemon juice (allow to stand 5–7 min.)
¼ cup onions or scallions	¼ cup chives or leeks *or* 1 tsp. onion powder
½ tsp. lemon juice	Just less than ¼ tsp. lemon extract or vinegar, to taste
Bananas, cherries, pineapple and other fruits not allowed	Use extracts or substitute strawberries
Canned tomato sauce	See Sauce Section p. 61 *or* Sugarless canned tomato sauce
Marinara sauce	See Sauce Section p. 56
Canned soups	See Soup Section p. 41
Bread crumbs	Gluten Bread Crumbs p. 143 *or* Equal amount of sunflower kernels, crushed in blender

When recipe calls for:	*Substitute:*
	until they are the texture of fine bread crumbs
White sauce	White Cream Sauce p. 55
Pastry crusts	See Dessert Section p. 113
Noodles, rice, spaghetti etc.	See Pasta Section p. 142
Frosting	See Cream Frosting p. 115
Gluten flour and bread (when used to thicken sauces and gravies)	Combine ingredients with water chestnuts in blender until desired consistency is obtained (about 6 nuts replace each slice of bread)

Many other substitutions may be found in this book. These are just a few of those called for most frequently.

Keep in Mind

Ketchup, sauces, canned or frozen fruits and vegetables are all assumed to be prepared without sugar unless listed otherwise on diet.

Use large eggs in recipes which call for eggs.

All recipes calling for sugar substitutes are written to allow choice of brand or type.

Imitation vanilla extract was used in all recipes calling for vanilla extract.

All baking should be done in pre-heated ovens unless otherwise indicated.

Steaming is the preferred method of vegetable preparation in all recipes calling for cooked vegetables.

Cook frozen vegetables while still frozen for all recipes in which they are used.

It would be well to reserve listed salt for use on cooked meats and vegetables except when drawing out of juices and flavor is desired for stews, soups, sauces and gravies.

M.S.G. (monosodium glutamate) has been included in some recipes for those who wish to use it. It is an optional ingredient.

Part Two

Recipes for the Strict Diet

Hors d'Oeuvres

Many of these hors d'oeuvres make excellent snack foods, especially those using generous amounts of cheese; they are high in protein and in taste appeal. Part of a batch of hors d'oeuvres may be eaten for a daytime snack, and part saved to be the appetizer before dinner.

FANCY STUFFED MUSHROOMS

12 lg. mushrooms
1 Tbsp. butter
1 clove garlic, crushed
2 Tbsp. parsley, chopped
For Liberal Diet, add 1 Tbsp. Gluten Bread Crumbs, p. 143.
2 tsp. basil or oregano
Pinch nutmeg
½ tsp. salt
¼ tsp. pepper
2 tsp. dry white wine
2 Tbsp. chives, chopped
¼ cup butter

Clean mushrooms and remove stems. Set caps aside and chop stems. Sauté stems in 1 Tbsp. butter for 2 min. or until they change color. Add garlic and cook 1 min. Add parsley, (Crumbs), basil, nutmeg, salt, pepper, wine and chives. In another pan, melt ¼ cup butter. Dip caps in butter and arrange in baking pan. Stuff with stem mixture and bake at 350 degrees for 15 min. Remove and broil to brown tops lightly.

Serves 4.

RUMAKI

Chicken livers
Water chestnuts
Bacon
Oil

Cut chicken livers in half. Slice water chestnuts leaving slices thick. Place 1 slice water chestnut between 2 halves of chicken liver, wrap in bacon slice and secure with a toothpick. Deep fry for approximately 3 min. Remove, drain and serve.

NORMA'S CAPONATA DELUXE

1 med. eggplant
½ cup olive oil
2 Tbsp. olive oil
1¼ cups chives, chopped fine
2 cups celery, sliced thin
1 green pepper, diced
3 Tbsp. tomato paste
½ cup water
½ cup vinegar
Sugar substitute equivalent to 2 tsp. sugar
1 clove garlic, mashed
1 Tbsp. parsley, chopped
½ cup stuffed green olives
⅓ cup capers
Salt and pepper, to taste

Dice eggplant into 1-in. cubes and sauté in ½ cup oil for 10–15 min., stirring frequently. Remove eggplant from oil, add 2 Tbsp. oil and sauté chives, celery and pepper for 3 min. Add eggplant and remaining ingredients, cover and simmer over low heat for 10 min. (For Liberal Diet, serve with toasted gluten bread squares.)

Serves 6–8.

CHEESE-BEEF BALL FONDUE

1 lb. ground beef
1 egg, slightly beaten
½ cup Gluten Bread Crumbs (p. 143)
½ tsp. salt
¼ tsp. pepper
¼ tsp. garlic powder
3 oz. Swiss cheese, cut into ¼-in. cubes
4 cups beef bouillon
½ lb. whole mushrooms
½ lb. cherry tomatoes
3 med. green peppers, cut into squares
2 cups Avocado Sauce (p. 59), optional

Combine beef with egg, (Crumbs), salt, pepper and garlic powder. Shape into balls around cheese cubes. Heat bouillon in fondue pot. String meatballs, mushrooms, tomatoes and peppers onto skewers. Cook in boiling bouillon 3–4 min. Serve with Avocado Sauce, if desired.

Serves 8.

VERSATILE VEAL FONDUE

Oil
Salt and pepper
3–3½ lbs. veal cubes, trimmed (about 1 in. square)
2 cups Tomato-Cheese Sauce (p. 58)

Pour oil to fill half of fondue pot. Heat until oil is bubbling. Lightly season veal and place in serving bowl with fondue forks. Reduce heat slightly under oil and cook cubes by plunging them into oil. Use Tomato-Cheese Sauce as a dip.

Suggestions:
Use salad dressing assortment for dipping veal.
Any favorite sauce may replace Tomato-Cheese Sauce.
Beef or fish may be substituted for veal.

Serves 12.

SHRIMP-CRAB COCKTAIL

- ½ lb. shrimp
- ½ lb. crab, flaked
- 3½ cups Seafood Sauce Marvel (p. 60) (May add extra ketchup to soften flavor.)
- 6 lemon wedges

Combine shrimp, crab and Seafood Sauce Marvel. Spoon into appetizer cups. Garnish with lemon wedges.

Makes about 6 generous cocktails.

FRESH VEGETABLE DIP

- ¾ cup mayonnaise
- ¾ cup sour cream
- 1 tsp. dill weed
- 4 tsp. dehydrated parsley flakes
- ¼–½ tsp. onion powder

Mix mayonnaise and sour cream together. Add remaining ingredients and refrigerate overnight. Serve with celery sticks, bell pepper wedges and pieces of cauliflower.

Makes 1½ cups.

CHEESE-CLAM DIP

- 2 Tbsp. mayonnaise
- 1 cup cream cheese, softened
- 1 (6½ oz.) can clams, drained and minced
- ¼ tsp. onion powder
- 2 tsp. black olives, chopped
- 1½ tsp. steak sauce
- Salt and pepper, to taste

Cream mayonnaise and cheese together. Add remaining ingredients.

Makes 1½ cups.

DIP GOURMET

2 cups mayonnaise
2 cups small curd cottage cheese
½ tsp. salt
½ cup chives, chopped
¼ tsp. hot pepper sauce (Tabasco)
¼ tsp. garlic powder
½ tsp. celery seeds
1 tsp. caraway seeds
1½ Tbsp. Worcestershire sauce
1 tsp. dry mustard
1 tsp. pepper

Combine all ingredients in mixing bowl. Chill and serve surrounded by mild white cheese slices.

Variation: This versatile dip may also be served with fresh-cut vegetables.

Makes 4 cups.

CHILI CON QUESO

2 lbs. cheddar cheese
1 (1 lb., 12 oz.) can whole tomatoes
3 Tbsp. Salsa Jalapeña (hot red chili relish)

Cut cheese into small chunks. Drain tomatoes, retaining liquid, and mash as they heat in a saucepan. Meanwhile, bring water to boil in double boiler and reduce heat. Pour hot mashed tomatoes into top of boiler, add cheese and chili relish. Simmer 30 min. If mixture becomes too thick, add small amount of retained liquid. Serve in a chafing dish with vegetables. (For Liberal Diet, serve with pieces of baked taco shells or small squares of toasted gluten bread.)

Cooking Hints: This dish may be made over direct heat, but constant stirring and very slow heat are required to prevent sticking. Use wooden spoon when stirring melted cheeses.

Serves 8–10.

CHILI CHEESE BALL

1 lb. cheddar cheese, grated
½ cup green chilies, diced
⅓ cup olives, diced fine
¼ cup parsley, chopped fine

Mix cheese with chilies and olives. Form into a ball and chill. Roll ball in parsley before serving.

Serves 6.

CHILI BEEF ROLLS

½ cup cottage cheese
1 Tbsp. chili sauce
¼ tsp. Worcestershire sauce
Salt and pepper, to taste
6 slices roast beef, cooked

Mix cottage cheese, chili sauce, Worcestershire sauce, salt and pepper. Spread on beef slices. Roll and secure with toothpicks.

Suggestion: Use these for snacks.

Makes 6 rolls.

CARAWAY CHEESE ROUNDS

3 oz. cream cheese
2 Tbsp. dill pickles, minced
¼ tsp. caraway seeds
Salt, to taste
1 hard-boiled egg
1 Tbsp. parsley, minced

Combine cream cheese, pickles, seeds and salt. Flatten, cut into rounds and chill. Push egg through sieve and mix with parsley. Cover rounds on both sides with egg mixture.

Makes 12 1-in. rounds.

CREAM CHEESE AND AVOCADO DIP

2 lg. avocados
8 oz. cream cheese, softened
½ cup mayonnaise
¼ cup lemon juice
1½ cups chives, chopped
Dash Worcestershire sauce
Salt, to taste

Combine all ingredients and serve with fresh vegetables cut to dipping size.

Serves 10.

BLEU CHEESE BALLS WITH ALMONDS

2 oz. bleu cheese, softened
2 oz. smoked cheese, softened
4 oz. cream cheese, softened
1 Tbsp. pimiento, chopped fine
1 Tbsp. green pepper, chopped fine
⅛ tsp. garlic powder
Dash salt
½ cup almonds, chopped

Cream cheeses together with a fork. Add pimiento, pepper, garlic powder and salt. Form into balls and roll in almonds.

Makes 16.

Eggs

Fill omelet with strawberries and top with strawberries and sour cream.

Scramble 4 eggs with 1 can shrimp. Add chives for flavor.

Scramble 4 eggs with ½ cup cottage cheese.

Make Tangy Omelet (p. 33) with crab meat or tuna.

Top eggs with Hollandaise Sauce (p. 57).

Fill omelet with ham bits and Swiss cheese.

Top favorite style eggs with Cream of Mushroom Soup (p. 46) or Cream of Tomato Soup (p. 44).

Pour clam sauce over eggs.

Flake any leftover fish into omelet and cover with Tomato Sauce (p. 61).

STRAWBERRY OMELET SOUFFLÉ

- 6 eggs, separated
- ½ tsp. salt
- 1 tsp. vanilla extract
- Sugar substitute equivalent to 3 Tbsp. sugar
- 2 tsp. lemon rind, grated
- 4 Tbsp. butter
- 1 lb. strawberries

Beat egg whites with salt until stiff peaks form. Beat yolks with vanilla, sugar substitute and lemon rind. Fold into egg whites. Melt butter in pan and pour in egg mixture. Brown lightly. Fill half of omelet with strawberries and fold in half. Slide onto serving plate and top with additional strawberries.

Serves 4–6.

TANGY OMELET

2 eggs
1 Tbsp. light cream
¼ tsp. Tabasco sauce
Salt and pepper, to taste
Butter

Beat eggs with cream, Tabasco, salt and pepper until frothy. Melt butter in pan and pour in egg mixture. Rotate pan in circular motion until mixture sets. When lightly browned, fold and slide onto platter.

Serves 1.

OMELET REJOICE

2 eggs
2 Tbsp. light cream
Salt and pepper, as desired
Butter
Cheddar cheese slices
3 strips bacon, cooked and crumbled
⅓ cup tomatoes, diced

Beat eggs with cream, salt and pepper until frothy. Melt butter in pan and pour in egg mixture. Rotate pan in circular motion until mixture sets. Cover half of omelet with cheese slices. Sprinkle bacon over cheese. Add tomatoes. When omelet is lightly browned, fold. Remove to serving platter.

Variations:
Add green peppers or mushrooms over cheese.
For Liberal Diet, add ¼ cup chopped onion.

Serves 1.

EGGS BENEDICT WITH CRAB SAUCE

1¼ cups Cream of Mushroom Soup (p. 46)
Dash Tabasco
2½ Tbsp. tomato paste
2 (7¾ oz.) cans king crab meat, drained with membranes removed, flaked
For Liberal Diet, add gluten toast, if desired.
6 eggs, poached

Heat Cream of Mushroom Soup with Tabasco and tomato paste. Add crab meat. Do not allow to boil. Place eggs on plate (or toast) and cover with crab sauce.

Serves 4–6.

CREAM CHEESE EGG SCRAMBLE

2 eggs
1 tsp. light cream
Salt, as desired
3 oz. cream cheese, softened
2–3 Tbsp. butter
1 med. tomato, diced or sliced

Beat eggs with cream and salt. Cut cream cheese into small cubes and add to eggs. Melt butter in pan and add egg mixture. Mash cream cheese while scrambling eggs. Stir constantly to prevent sticking. Toss in tomatoes just before removing from heat. Serve immediately.

Serves 1.

POACHED EGGS MARINARA

4 eggs
2 slices Swiss cheese, cut to fit over eggs
1 cup Marinara Sauce (p. 56)
6 slices bacon, cooked and crumbled

Poach eggs with cheese. Remove to serving platter, spoon Marinara Sauce over eggs and top with bacon.

Serves 2.

COTTAGE SCRAMBLED EGGS

6 eggs
½ cup, half light cream, half water
For Liberal Diet, substitute ½ cup milk.
½ tsp. salt
¼ tsp. pepper
1 cup cottage cheese
3 Tbsp. butter
2 tomatoes, sliced

Beat eggs with cream, salt and pepper. Fold in cottage cheese and scramble in butter, stirring constantly. Serve over tomato slices.

Serves 4.

MUSHROOM POACHED EGGS WITH SOUR CREAM

4 eggs, poached
1 (4 oz.) can mushrooms, sautéed in butter
1 cup sour cream
Salt and pepper, to taste
½ cup sharp cheddar cheese, grated

Place eggs in baking dish. Cover each with mushrooms and ¼ of sour cream. Season with salt and pepper; top with cheese. Bake at 375 degrees until cheese melts. Serve immediately.

Serves 2–4.

SCRAMBLED EGG BAKE

6 eggs
¾ cup, half light cream, half water
For Liberal Diet, substitute ¾ cup milk.
Salt and pepper, as desired
Parsley, chopped fine

Beat eggs slightly with cream, salt and pepper. Pour into well-buttered 8-in. square baking pan. Place in larger pan of hot water and bake at 350 degrees for 25–30 min. Eggs may be stirred before serving. Sprinkle with parsley.

Serves 3.

LATIN EGG DELIGHT

2 Tbsp. oil
1 clove garlic, minced
¾ cup chives, chopped
1 sm. green pepper, chopped
½ tsp. marjoram
¼ tsp. cayenne
1 cup Basic Tomato Sauce (p. 61)
1 (1 lb.) can tomatoes, drained and chopped
Salt and pepper, to taste
6 eggs

Heat oil and sauté garlic, chives and green pepper until tender. Add marjoram, cayenne, Tomato Sauce and tomatoes. Cook until sauce comes to a boil. Lower heat, add salt and pepper. Drop eggs into sauce and simmer, covered, until eggs are set. Serve eggs with sauce spooned over top.

Serves 4–6.

GREEN PEPPER EGG BAKE

2½ Tbsp. green pepper, chopped
2½ Tbsp. chives, chopped
2 Tbsp. butter
1 pt. cottage cheese
6 eggs
Salt, to taste
Parsley, chopped

Sauté green pepper and chives in butter until tender. Mix with cottage cheese. Form nests in well-buttered baking dish. Open 1 egg into each, salt and sprinkle with parsley. Bake at 325 degrees for 12–15 min. or until eggs are done.

Serves 4–6.

CANADIAN EGGS

4 slices sharp cheddar cheese
8 slices Canadian bacon, cooked
4 eggs
2 Tbsp. light cream
Salt and pepper, to taste
2 Tbsp. parsley
Butter

Melt 1 slice of cheese on each 2 pieces of bacon. Beat eggs with cream, salt, pepper and parsley. Scramble in butter and place mounds of eggs over cheese.

Serves 4.

STUFFED EGGS

Suggestions for fillings:
Use tuna or salmon with curry powder.
Mix ham or bacon bits with garlic powder.
Stuff with sardines and tomato bits.
Mix yolks with anchovy fillets, capers and pimiento.
Stuff with any leftover meats and spices.

AVOCADO STUFFED EGGS

6 hard-boiled eggs, cut in half lengthwise
½ med. avocado, peeled and chopped
⅛ tsp. cayenne
1 Tbsp. dehydrated parsley flakes
¾ tsp. lemon juice
½ tsp. salt
Pinch onion powder

Remove egg yolks and mix them with remaining ingredients. Stuff mixture back into whites.

CHEESE STUFFED EGGS

4 hard-boiled eggs, cut in half lengthwise
2 Tbsp. sharp cheddar cheese, crumbled
¼ cup cream cheese, softened
2 tsp. dehydrated parsley flakes
Paprika, for garnish

Remove egg yolks and mix them with remaining ingredients. Stuff mixture back into whites and garnish with paprika, if desired.

TURKEY STUFFED EGGS

¼ cup celery, chopped
⅓ cup mayonnaise
⅛ tsp. salt
½ cup turkey, diced small
¼ tsp. dry mustard
6 hard-boiled eggs, cut in half lengthwise
Paprika

Combine celery, mayonnaise, salt, turkey and mustard with egg yolks. Stuff mixture back into whites and garnish with paprika.

Variation: Substitute chicken for turkey.

LOBSTER STUFFED EGGS

½ cup lobster bits
¼ tsp. salt
Pinch pepper
¼ cup mayonnaise
¼ cup green pepper, chopped fine
4 hard-boiled eggs, cut in half lengthwise
Parmesan cheese

Mix lobster with salt, pepper, mayonnaise, green pepper and egg yolks. Stuff back into whites and garnish with Parmesan cheese.

Variations: Use crab meat instead of lobster.

BREAKFAST PUFFS

1 egg white
Sugar substitute equivalent to 2 tsp. sugar
1 egg yolk beaten with dash salt
⅛ tsp. baking soda
⅛ tsp. vanilla extract
1 Tbsp. light cream
3 Tbsp. ricotta cheese
Butter

Beat egg white with sugar substitute and refrigerate. Combine all remaining ingredients except butter, and fold into chilled white. Drop by teaspoonfuls onto hot buttered pan. Cook until center is dry. (These rise like little cakes when baked at 350 degrees on a cookie sheet.)

Serves 1–2.

BLINTZ OMELETS

3 eggs
3 tsp. light cream
Dash salt
Butter
Filling for Cheese Blintzes (p. 178)

Beat each egg with 1 tsp. cream and a dash salt. Heat butter in pan. Pour 1 egg into pan and rotate until egg sets. Drop ⅓ of Filling, by tablespoonfuls, onto half of egg. Fold omelet in half and continue cooking until done as desired.

Suggestion: Serve with sour cream.

Makes 3 omelets.

Soups

You need not abandon soups or favorite recipes which have soup as an ingredient. The soup recipes below are flavorful and easy to prepare. Cream soups can double as sauces for vegetables and meats.

One egg per recipe may be added to most of the soups. While this increases the protein content it does not change the soup itself. Chicken broth may be substituted for water or milk in most recipes with delightful results.

Combine soups for welcome changes in flavor. For example, using tomato soup as a base, mix with Cream of Mushroom or Onion or Cream of Celery or Green Pea.

Be imaginative and create soups of your own. As a guide, use two cups White Cream Sauce to one cup vegetables and add spices to taste. Soups may be thickened by adding gluten or soya flour, 1 Tbsp. at a time, until desired consistency is achieved.

Recipes using White Cream Sauce are much easier to handle if prepared in a double boiler because this sauce should never be allowed to boil. I have provided directions for preparation in a saucepan in case a double boiler is not available.

CREAM OF CLAM SOUP

1 cup clams, minced, with juice
2 cups White Cream Sauce (p. 55)
¼ tsp. paprika
Dash Worcestershire sauce
Dash oregano
½ tsp. salt
¼ tsp. white pepper

Process all ingredients in blender until smooth. Heat slowly. Do not allow to boil.

Serves 2–3.

SHRIMP CURRY SOUP

1 cup, half light cream, half water
For Liberal Diet, substitute 1 cup milk.
1 (4½ oz.) can shrimp and liquid
2 tsp. dehydrated parsley flakes
¼ cup green pepper, diced
1 tsp. onion powder
¾ tsp. salt
½ tsp. curry powder
Dash Tabasco sauce
1 cup Cream of Mushroom Soup (p. 46)

Combine cream, shrimp and liquid, parsley flakes, green pepper, onion powder, salt, curry powder and Tabasco in blender until smooth. Pour into saucepan and add Mushroom Soup. Stir and heat slowly until hot and soup is of desired thickness. Do not allow to boil.

Serves 4.

FRESH TOMATO SOUP

¾ tsp. onion powder
For Liberal Diet, substitute 3 Tbsp. onion, diced.
1½ tsp. salt
Sugar substitute equivalent to 2 tsp. sugar
1 cup water
1½ Tbsp. butter
Dash Tabasco sauce
Dash pepper
1 (1 lb., 12 oz.) can whole tomatoes and liquid

In blender container, combine onion powder, salt, sugar substitute, water, butter, Tabasco and pepper. Process until smooth. Remove to a saucepan. Pour tomatoes and liquid into blender container and process slowly until liquefied.

Pour into saucepan through a sieve (to remove seeds). Heat, stirring occasionally, until soup is desired thickness (usually 20–25 min.).

Makes about 4 servings.

HOMEMADE VEGETABLE-BEEF SOUP

- 5 lb. chuck roast
- 2 tsp. onion powder
- 12 oz. tomato paste
- ½ tsp. Worcestershire sauce
- 2 Tbsp. dehydrated parsley flakes
- ¼ tsp. garlic powder
- ¼ tsp. sage
- ½ tsp. Parmesan cheese, grated
- ¼ tsp. Tabasco sauce
- Sugar substitute equivalent to 2 tsp. sugar
- 1 cup celery, diced
- ½ tsp. lemon juice
- ½ cup bell pepper, diced
- 2 (1 lb., 12 oz.) cans whole tomatoes and liquid
- 1 cup spinach, chopped
- ½ cup zucchini, chopped
- 3 cups any allowed vegetable, cut bite size
- Salt, pepper, garlic salt, as desired

Season meat and place in large soup pot. Cover with water and add onion powder. Bring water to a boil, reduce heat and cover. Simmer for 1½ hrs. Cool and remove fat layer. Remove meat, trim and cut into small pieces. Return to pot with 9 cups of the liquid. Heat and add all remaining ingredients. Simmer, covered, until all vegetables are soft and soup has thickened, about 1 hr.

Makes 6–8 quarts.

CREAM OF TOMATO SOUP

2 cups White Cream Sauce (p. 55)
1 cup fresh tomatoes
3½ Tbsp. bell pepper, chopped
½ tsp. dehyrdrated parsley flakes
⅛ tsp. onion powder

Process all ingredients in blender until smooth. Cook over low heat until hot. Do not allow to boil. Serve immediately. *Suggestion:* Try floating bacon bits on top of each serving.

Makes 2 cups.

MUSHROOM BISQUE WITH SOUR CREAM CAPS

1 lb. sm. mushrooms
4 cups chicken broth
4 Tbsp. butter
¼ tsp. dry mustard
Pinch nutmeg
1 egg white, beaten until peaks form
¼ cup dry red wine
½ cup cream
Sour cream and paprika, if desired for garnish

Wash mushrooms and remove stems. Add chopped stems to chicken broth and simmer for 25 min. Strain broth and set aside. Sauté caps in butter until light brown. Mix mustard and nutmeg. Stir mixture in with caps. Slowly add broth and egg white. Stir over low heat for 8–10 min. Add wine and cream. Heat. Each serving may be topped with sour cream and sprinkled with paprika.

Serves 6–8.

CREAM OF ASPARAGUS SOUP

2 lb. asparagus, cooked and cut into pieces
2 cups White Cream Sauce (p. 55)
1 Tbsp. butter, soft
1¼ tsp. salt
½ tsp. pepper
½ tsp. onion powder
¼ tsp. celery salt
1 cup, half light cream, half water
For Liberal Diet, substitute 1 cup milk.
Sharp cheddar cheese, grated

Put cooked asparagus in blender and add remaining ingredients. Process until smooth. Heat but do not allow to boil. Float grated cheese on top of each serving.

Serves 4–6.

CREAM OF CELERY SOUP

3 cups White Cream Sauce (p. 55)
1½ cups celery, cooked and cut into pieces
2½ tsp. onion powder
For Liberal Diet, substitute ⅔ cup onions.
½ tsp. salt
¼ tsp. white pepper
1 Tbsp. dehydrated parsley flakes
1 bay leaf

Combine 1 cup White Cream Sauce with celery, onion powder, salt, pepper and parsley flakes in blender. Process until smooth. Pour into a saucepan and add remaining 2 cups White Cream Sauce. Place bay leaf on top and simmer 20 min. Remove bay leaf and serve.

Serves 4–6.

CREAM OF CHICKEN SOUP

18 water chestnuts
For Liberal Diet, substitute 3 slices gluten bread.
3 Tbsp. butter
½ tsp. salt
¼ tsp. pepper
1 cup heavy cream
For Liberal Diet, substitute 1 cup light cream.
1 cup chicken broth
¾ cup chicken, cooked and diced
½ tsp. onion powder

Combine all ingredients in blender and process until smooth. Heat and serve.

Makes 2 generous cups.

CREAM OF MUSHROOM SOUP

3 oz. sliced mushrooms
1½ tsp. celery, diced
Butter
1½ cups White Cream Sauce (p. 55)
Dash pepper
¼ tsp. onion powder
Chives

Sauté mushrooms and celery in butter. Add to White Cream Sauce with pepper and onion powder in blender. Process until smooth. Cook over low heat until hot, but do not allow to boil. Serve immediately. Sprinkle chives on top of each serving.

Makes 2 cups.

Salads and Dressings

Because recipes for various types of molds are so readily available, I have purposely not included many. Your favorite molds from pre-diet days may be adapted easily by using unflavored gelatin or flavored diet ones in place of regular flavors containing sugar. Do not overlook the value of this type of salad. With a minimum of effort you can produce a dish that is delicious and high in protein.*

Make seafood molds often. They are an excellent addition to a meal and leftovers make outstanding snacks. Green salads can be made more interesting and nutritious by using a good selection of vegetables. Escarole, bean sprouts and spinach add flavor and texture to an otherwise ordinary salad.

Use bacon bits and grated Parmesan cheese liberally in tossed salads to increase appeal as well as protein content. Avocado gives salad new life and is extremely healthful. If you are on the Strict Diet, toss in a few chives for that onion flavor you may miss.

Some good salad dressings acceptable on this diet are available commercially. Should you prefer homemade dressing, some excellent ones appear in this section. Also it's quite easy to adjust recipes for other dressings by making use of the Substitutions List on p. 20.

There is no excuse for a dull salad!

* Gelatin does not contain all of the essential amino acids. It provides usable protein when prepared with eggs or eaten with a source of complete protein.

TANGY TUNA SALAD

½ cup cucumber, diced
¼ cup green pepper, chopped
1 can tuna, flaked
⅓ cup mayonnaise
¼ cup ketchup
2 tsp. taco sauce
Salt and pepper, to taste

Mix cucumber and green pepper with tuna. Combine mayonnaise, ketchup and taco sauce. Pour over tuna mixture. Mix and season with salt and pepper.

Suggestions:

Stuff tuna mixture into tomato shells and top with chopped parsley.

For Liberal Diet, stuff tuna mixture into cleaned green peppers and top with Buttered Gluten Bread Crumbs.

Serves 2.

CHEESY ORANGE GEL

1 envelope orange diet gelatin
½ cup hot water
1 cup cold water
Sugar substitute, to taste
½ cup cottage cheese
½ cup sour cream
For Liberal Diet, add 1 (4 oz.) can mandarin orange segments, drained.

Dissolve gelatin in hot water and add cold. Sweeten and refrigerate until mixture is the consistency of egg whites. Combine cottage cheese, sour cream (and orange segments). Stir into gelatin mixture and refrigerate until firm.

Serves 4.

BEST SALMON MOUSSE

2 cups salmon, cooked and flaked
½ cup mayonnaise
1 cup cottage cheese, beaten smooth
½ cup light cream
⅛ tsp. onion powder
Dash Tabasco sauce
1½ tsp. capers, chopped
½ tsp. salt
¼ tsp. pepper
1 envelope unflavored gelatin
¼ cup cold water
1½ cups hot water

Mix salmon, mayonnaise, cottage cheese, cream, onion powder, Tabasco, capers, salt and pepper. Soften gelatin in cold water and dissolve in hot according to package directions. Cool slightly and stir into salmon mixture. Place in oiled 1½-qt. mold. Chill until firm.

Note: Fish molds—tuna, shrimp, for instance—are excellent sources of protein and can be extremely tasty. A great variety of such recipes are available in regular cookbooks.

Serves 6.

COTTAGE STRAWBERRY SALAD

1½ cups strawberries
1½ cups cottage cheese
1½ cups sour cream
Sugar substitute, to taste
Lettuce

Slice strawberries. Mix with cottage cheese and sour cream. Sweeten to taste. Spoon onto lettuce beds.

Serves 4.

AVOCADO-COTTAGE LOAF

1 envelope lemon-flavored diet gelatin
½ cup hot water
1 cup cold water
¾ medium avocado
½ cup cottage cheese
⅓ cup chives, chopped
⅓ cup sour cream

Dissolve gelatin in hot water and dilute with cold. Chill until slightly thickened. Mash avocado into cottage cheese. Add chives and sour cream. Mix into gelatin and pour into mold. Chill until set.

Serves 4.

EXALTED CAESAR SALAD

1 clove garlic
½ cup salad oil
1 head romaine
4 tomatoes, diced
1 (2 oz.) can anchovy fillets, drained
½ tsp. salt
½ tsp. pepper
¼ cup lemon juice
1 egg
½ cup Parmesan cheese, grated
For Liberal Diet, add 1 cup Croutons Parmesan (p. 144).

Mash garlic into oil. Strain to remove garlic. Set aside. Wash romaine and break into bite-size pieces. Add tomatoes and anchovies. Sprinkle oil over salad and toss with fork and spoon until greens are glistening. Combine salt, pepper, lemon juice and egg. Beat well and add cheese. Pour dressing over top. (Add Croutons Parmesan.) Toss lightly.

Serves 4–6.

BLEU CHEESE DRESSING

- 6 oz. bleu cheese, crumbled
- 1 cup sour cream
- 8 oz. cream cheese
- ½ cup + 2 Tbsp. cream
- Garlic powder, to taste
- Dash salt
- 1¾ cups mayonnaise

Combine all ingredients well and refrigerate.

Variation: Substitute Roquefort cheese for bleu cheese.

Makes 5 cups.

AVOCADO DRESSING

- 1 med. avocado, peeled and pitted
- 2 Tbsp. mayonnaise
- ¼ tsp. salt
- ⅓ cup water
- ¾ tsp. lemon juice
- Dash onion powder
- Dash pepper
- ¼ tsp. Salsa Jalapeña (hot red chili relish)

Combine all ingredients in blender until smooth. Chill.

Makes about 1 cup.

ROMANO SALAD DRESSING

- ½ cup mayonnaise
- 2 Tbsp. oil
- 2 Tbsp. vinegar
- 6 Tbsp. Romano cheese, grated
- Garlic powder, to taste

Combine all ingredients and mix well. Chill and serve over salad.

Makes 1 cup.

ZINGY ITALIAN DRESSING

½ tsp. dry mustard
½ tsp. pepper
1½ tsp. salt
1¼ tsp. paprika
Sugar substitute equivalent to ¾ tsp. sugar
¾ cup vinegar
1½ cups salad oil

Mix all ingredients well and chill.

Suggestions:

This dressing is an exceptional marinade for vegetables.

Use on chicken or turkey salads, also brush it on before cooking.

Makes about 2 cups.

SPICY THOUSAND ISLAND DRESSING

½ cup mayonnaise
2 Tbsp. ketchup
½ sm. dill pickle, chopped fine
3 drops taco sauce (may substitute Tabasco)
Dash salt, pepper, onion powder and M.S.G. (monosodium glutamate)
⅛ tsp. white vinegar or lemon juice

Combine all ingredients. Chill and store in jar with tight-fitting lid.

Makes about 1½ cups.

Sauces, Syrups, Jellies and Jams

One outstanding sauce can transform any ordinary dish into a gourmet's delight. I have included many such sauces in this section. Use them to transform meals into special occasions.

The White Cream Sauce serves many purposes. It is not only used as a white sauce substitute, but also as a basic recipe for creating other sauces and soups.

Cheese sauces are versatile. Take full advantage of their protein content and aesthetic appeal.

The Ginger Sauce is our family favorite. Everyone enjoys it spooned over Poppy Seed Chicken (p. 104). I often serve it to guests, too.

GINGER SAUCE

15–18 water chestnuts
For Liberal Diet, substitute 3 slices gluten bread.
3 Tbsp. butter
1½ cups chicken broth
½ tsp. salt
¼ tsp. pepper
½ tsp. ginger

Mix all ingredients in blender container until smooth. Heat in double boiler or in saucepan over low heat, stirring often. Serve immediately.

Suggestion: Delicious over chicken and seafood.

Makes about 1¾ cups.

NUTMEG SAUCE

Substitute nutmeg for ginger and follow directions for Ginger Sauce (above).

TARTAR SAUCE

- 1½ Tbsp. salad peppers, in jar
- 1 cup mayonnaise
- 1 tsp. liquid from salad peppers
- ¼ tsp. garlic powder
- ⅛ tsp. onion powder

Remove stems from salad peppers. Slit open, remove seeds and chop. Combine peppers with all remaining ingredients and chill.

Makes 1 cup.

TOMATO-CLAM SAUCE

- ⅔ cup chives, chopped fine
  For Liberal Diet, substitute ⅔ cup scallions.
- 2 Tbsp. butter
- ¾ tsp. garlic powder
- ¾ tsp. oregano
- ½ cup dry white wine
- ½ cup heavy cream
- 1½ Tbsp. parsley flakes
- 1 tsp. salt
- ⅛ tsp. pepper
- 1 (1 lb., 12 oz.) can tomatoes, drained
- 1 (8 oz.) can minced clams
  Liquid from clams

Sauté chives in butter. Add garlic powder, oregano, wine, cream, parsley flakes, salt and pepper. Add tomatoes and mash. Simmer 5–7 min. Add clams and liquid. Simmer for an additional 4–5 min. and serve.

Suggestions for Liberal Diet:
Spoon over Cheese-Tomato Pizza.
Mix with Gluten Linguine and serve as side dish.
Use as spaghetti sauce.

Makes about 2½ cups.

WHITE CREAM SAUCE

5–6 water chestnuts
For Liberal Diet, substitute 1 slice gluten bread.
2 Tbsp. butter
¼ tsp. salt
⅛ tsp. pepper
1 cup light cream
Dash cream of tartar

Place water chestnuts (bread) in blender and add remaining ingredients. Process until mixed thoroughly (bread is crumbled). Heat in double boiler (or saucepan, stirring constantly), until smooth and thickened.

For medium sauce, add 10–12 water chestnuts (2 slices of bread).

Add 15–18 water chestnuts (3 slices) for thick sauce.

Suggestion: For instant White Cream Sauce, substitute 1 cup hot cream for cold, and blend. Serve without cooking.

Makes 1 generous cup.

LEMON CREAM SAUCE WITH BUTTON MUSHROOMS

1 cup White Cream Sauce (above)
½ tsp. lemon juice
¼ tsp. onion powder
½ tsp. parsley flakes
Dash salt
⅛ tsp. paprika
1 small can button mushrooms

Combine all ingredients except mushrooms and mix in blender. Add mushrooms and heat gently. Serve over chops and steaks.

Makes 1½ cups.

MARINARA SAUCE

1 cup chives, chopped
For Liberal Diet, substitute 1 cup onions.
2 cloves garlic, minced
3 Tbsp. butter
1 (1 lb.) can whole tomatoes
2 cups Basic Tomato Sauce (p. 61)
1½ tsp. basil
1½ tsp. thyme
¼ tsp. pepper
½ tsp. salt
Dash oregano, optional

Sauté chives and garlic in butter. Add tomatoes, Tomato Sauce, basil, thyme, pepper, salt and oregano. Cover and simmer 12–15 min.

Suggestions:

Put all ingredients, except butter, in blender and process until smooth. Heat and serve.

Use Marinara Sauce over breaded veal cutlets, chicken or seafood. Melt mozzarella cheese on top.

Makes 2½–3 cups.

DILL SAUCE

1½ cups sour cream
1 tsp. dill weed
2 Tbsp. chives, chopped fine
3 Tbsp. lemon juice
1 egg
Salt and pepper, as desired

Combine sour cream, dill weed, chives and lemon juice. Beat egg well and mix with sauce. Season with salt and pepper. Chill.

Suggestion: Slightly heat sauce to enhance flavor.

Makes about 2 cups.

ITALIAN SPAGHETTI SAUCE

1 (1 lb., 12 oz.) can Italian-style tomatoes, drained
⅓ cup liquid from canned tomatoes
½ cup tomato paste
5 Tbsp. bell pepper, diced
2 tsp. mushrooms
¼–½ tsp. onion powder
For Liberal Diet, substitute 2 Tbsp. onions.
½ tsp. parsley flakes
¾ tsp. garlic powder
¼ tsp. oregano
Dash Tabasco sauce
¼ tsp. salt
½ cup dry white wine
1 bay leaf

Blend all ingredients, except wine and bay leaf, in blender container until smooth. Add wine, stir and pour into a saucepan. Place bay leaf on top and simmer over low heat for 20 min. Remove bay leaf and serve.

Makes 4½ cups.

HOLLANDAISE SAUCE

3 egg yolks
3 Tbsp. lemon juice
½ cup butter

Place egg yolks, lemon juice and cut-up butter in top of double boiler. Allow to stand at room temperature for 30 min. Bring water to a gentle boil and place mixture over it. Stir constantly until mixture thickens, about 1½ min. Use immediately.

Makes ⅔ cup.

CHEESE SAUCE

5–6 water chestnuts
For Liberal Diet, substitute 1 slice gluten bread.
¼ tsp. salt
⅛ tsp. pepper
2 Tbsp. butter
½ cup cheddar cheese chunks
1 cup hot cream
For Liberal Diet, substitute 1 cup hot milk.

Put all ingredients in blender, adding cream last. Process until smooth.

Makes 1½ cups.

TOMATO-CHEESE SAUCE

2 Tbsp. fresh tomato, diced
½ tsp. parsley flakes
1/16 tsp. onion powder
1 cup Cheese Sauce (above)

Remove seeds from tomatoes. Blend all ingredients in blender until smooth and mixed thoroughly.

Makes 1 cup.

GARLIC CHEESE SAUCE

1 cup Cheese Sauce (above)
⅛ tsp. garlic powder
½ bay leaf

Process in blender until completely mixed and bay leaf is in very small bits.

Makes 1 cup.

SWISS CHEESE SAUCE

½ cup Swiss cheese chunks
5–6 water chestnuts
For Liberal Diet, substitute 1 slice gluten bread.
¼ tsp. salt
⅛ tsp. white pepper
1 cup, half light cream, half water, hot
For Liberal Diet, substitute 1 cup milk.

Combine all ingredients in blender, adding cream last. Process until smooth.

Makes 1½ cups.

AVOCADO SAUCE

2 Tbsp. sour cream
½ tsp. onion powder
For Liberal Diet, substitute 2 Tbsp. onion, diced.
5 Tbsp. water
¼ tsp. salt
Dash pepper
½ tsp. lemon juice
1/16 tsp. garlic powder
¾ tsp. Salsa Jalapeña (hot red chili relish)
1 med. avocado, peeled

Combine all ingredients in blender until smooth.

Makes about 2 cups.

HOT MUSTARD SAUCE

1 (9 oz.) jar mustard
3 Tbsp. horseradish
Dash Tabasco sauce

Mix and chill. Serve with beef dishes.

Makes 1 generous cup.

SESAME CREAMED MUSTARD

1 cup sour cream
¼ tsp. lemon juice
3–4 Tbsp. prepared mustard
½ tsp. sesame seeds

Mix and chill. Delicious with leg of lamb.

Makes 1 cup.

SEAFOOD SAUCE MARVEL

1 cup ketchup
½ tsp. onion powder
For Liberal Diet, substitute 2 Tbsp. onion, grated.
1 tsp. horseradish
½ tsp. lemon juice
⅛ tsp. salt
⅛ tsp. pepper
Sugar substitute equivalent to 2 tsp. sugar
¼ tsp. Worcestershire sauce
⅛ tsp. Tabasco sauce

Combine all ingredients, chill and serve.

Makes about 1¾ cups.

CLAM SAUCE

2 cloves garlic, minced
1 cup chives, chopped
For Liberal Diet, substitute 1 cup onions.
3 Tbsp. butter
1 (10 oz.) can whole clams with liquid
1¾ Tbsp. parsley, chopped
Salt and pepper, to taste

Sauté garlic and chives in butter. Add clams, liquid, parsley, salt and pepper. Simmer 4–5 min.

Suggestion: For Liberal Diet, serve over Gluten Linguine and sprinkle with grated Parmesan cheese.

Serves 2–4.

BASIC TOMATO SAUCE

1 (1 lb., 12 oz.) can whole tomatoes
1/3 cup liquid from canned tomatoes
1/2 cup tomato paste
1/4 cup bell pepper, diced
1/4–1/2 tsp. onion powder
For Liberal Diet, substitute 1 1/2 *Tbsp. onions.*
1/4 tsp. dehydrated parsley flakes
1/16 tsp. Tabasco sauce
1/4 tsp. salt

Drain tomatoes reserving required liquid. Process all ingredients in blender until smooth. Refrigerate in jar with tight-fitting lid. This sauce keeps well for several weeks.

Makes 3 3/4 cups.

TANGY RUM SAUCE

2 tsp. lemon juice
Sugar substitute equivalent to 2/3 cup sugar
4 egg yolks
1/3 cup dry white wine
1 cup heavy cream
3 Tbsp. light rum

Beat lemon juice, sugar substitute and egg yolks well. Remove mixture to top of double boiler and heat, stirring constantly. Add wine and continue cooking until sauce thickens. Remove to bowl. Whip cream with rum and fold into cooked mixture. Chill.

Makes 2 cups.

BRANDY SAUCE

Prepare Rum Sauce (p. 61), substituting brandy for rum.

MAPLE SYRUP

1 envelope unflavored gelatin
½ cup cold water
Sugar substitute equivalent to 1 cup sugar
1 tsp. maple flavoring
1½ cups boiling water

Dissolve gelatin in cold water according to package directions. Add sugar substitute and maple flavoring. Stir in boiling water and simmer for 3 min., stirring constantly. Refrigerate until mixture thickens and becomes desired consistency. If syrup becomes too thick, stir while container stands in hot water.

Makes 2 cups.

MAPLE-BUTTER SYRUP

Follow directions for Maple Syrup (above), adding 1 tsp. melted butter before simmering.

STRAWBERRY SYRUP

1 envelope unflavored gelatin
½ cup cold water
1 tsp. strawberry flavoring
Sugar substitute equivalent to 1 cup sugar
2 drops red food coloring
1½ cups boiling water

Soften gelatin in ½ cup cold water. Add strawberry flavoring, sugar substitute and food coloring. Stir in boiling water and simmer 3 min. Refrigerate until syrupy and cooled to room temperature. If syrup becomes too thick, stir while container sits in hot water until desired consistency.

Makes 2 cups.

RASPBERRY SYRUP

1 envelope raspberry diet gelatin
1 cup wild raspberry diet soda
⅛ tsp. imitation butter flavoring
1 tray ice cubes (12–14)
¼ cup cold water

Dissolve gelatin in boiling soda and add butter flavoring. Quickly stir in ice cubes. Stir until cubes no longer melt. Remove remaining pieces of ice. Add cold water, mix and pour into pitcher. Allow to stand at room temperature 5–10 min. or until mixture becomes syrupy. Serve over pancakes, crepes and desserts.

Variations: Substitute any favorite diet gelatin and mix with diet soda. Strawberry diet gelatin and black cherry diet drink make a delicious syrup.

Makes 2 cups.

STRAWBERRY JAM

1 pint strawberries, washed, with stems removed
¼ cup water
Sugar substitute equivalent to 2 cups sugar
1 Tbsp. lemon juice

Combine strawberries with water in a saucepan. Boil 2 min., stirring constantly. Add sugar substitute and continue boiling for an additional 2 min. Stir in lemon juice and remove to shallow pan. Allow to stand at room temperature for 8–10 hours, stirring occasionally. Put in jar with tight-fitting lid and refrigerate.

Variations: For Liberal Diet, substitute any allowed fruit for strawberries. Adjust sugar substitute to taste.

Makes about 1 cup.

STRAWBERRY JELLY-PRESERVES COMBO

1 envelope unflavored gelatin
⅓ cup cold water
1 can strawberry diet soda
Sugar substitute equivalent to ½ tsp. sugar
¼ tsp. imitation strawberry flavoring
6 medium strawberries, slightly mashed

Dissolve gelatin in cold water. Add remaining ingredients and simmer, stirring constantly, until jelly comes to a boil. Pour into jar, cool, cover with tight-fitting lid and refrigerate until jelly is slightly thickened and strawberries have settled to the bottom. Pour off clear jelly into another jar, seal and return to refrigerator, leaving preserves in original jar.

Suggestions:

Increase strawberries to 1½ cups for preserves.
Omit strawberries to make jelly.

Makes 2 cups.

Vegetables

Vegetables can be the most humdrum portion of your meal, but they need not be. Broiled, baked, fried, steamed and souffléed, prepared in a rich sauce or topped with a light one, vegetables are as versatile as your creativity allows.

With vegetables, use cheese and cheese sauces (found in Sauces Section) liberally. Add chopped nuts as a garnish to dress up ordinary recipes. These dishes do not have to be time-consuming and complicated to prepare for their flavor to be exceptional.

QUICKIE VEGETABLES

Stir ½ tsp. dry mustard into ¼ cup melted butter and serve over cooked cauliflower or cabbage.

Stir 1½ tsp. grated Romano cheese into ¼ cup melted butter and serve over broccoli, asparagus or brussels sprouts.

Stir ½ tsp. cayenne into ¼ cup melted butter and serve over spinach, cabbage or cauliflower.

Stir ½ tsp. onion powder and dash garlic powder into ¼ cup melted butter and serve over green beans, eggplant, string beans or broccoli.

Stir ½ tsp. basil and dash thyme into ¼ cup melted butter and serve over zucchini and green beans.

Stir ½ tsp. curry powder into ¼ cup melted butter and serve over string beans or spinach.

Use your imagination and favorite spices to create new flavor treats with vegetables. There is no excuse for serving them plain when they can be made unusual and delicious so easily!

BUSY DAY STEWED TOMATOES

1 (1 lb., 12 oz.) can whole tomatoes, with liquid
Sugar substitute equivalent to 1 tsp. sugar
¼ tsp. lemon juice
2 Tbsp. parsley flakes

Pour tomatoes and liquid into saucepan. Add sugar substitute, lemon juice and parsley flakes. Cover and simmer until heated thoroughly. Serve.

Serves 4.

STEWED TOMATOES MAGNIFIQUE

¼ cup bell pepper, diced
2 Tbsp. chives, minced
⅓ cup celery, minced
4 Tbsp. butter
1 (1 lb., 12 oz.) can whole tomatoes
Liquid from canned tomatoes, less ½ cup
½ cup tomato juice
¼ tsp. dehydrated parsley flakes
3 drops Worcestershire sauce
Sugar substitute equivalent to 1 tsp. sugar
¼ tsp. thyme
¼ tsp. salt
Dash oregano
Dash pepper
1 bay leaf

Sauté bell pepper, chives and celery in butter until they are soft. Cut tomatoes in half and spoon into a saucepan. Add liquid from can, tomato juice, parsley flakes, Worcestershire sauce, sweetener and spices. Mix well and put in sautéed vegetables. Place bay leaf on top and simmer about 10 min.

Serves 4.

CROWN CELERY

2 Tbsp. parsley, chopped
¾ cup green pepper, diced
4 cups celery, sliced thin
Salt, as desired
½ cup chicken broth
1 cup cottage cheese

Combine parsley, green pepper, celery, salt and broth in saucepan. Cook, uncovered, until celery is tender, about 20 min. Stir in cottage cheese. Simmer until hot, stirring often. Serve immediately.

Suggestion: For Liberal Diet, serve topped with Beet Vegetable Topping.

Serves 4–6.

BROCCOLI-CHEESE PARTY

1½ Tbsp. butter
½ cup sour cream
¼ cup sharp cheddar cheese, grated
1 (10 oz.) pkg. frozen chopped broccoli or ⅔ lb. fresh
¼ cup leeks, chopped
2 eggs
½ tsp. salt
¼ tsp. pepper
Pinch nutmeg
½ cup almonds, slivered

Melt butter and stir in sour cream and cheese. Add broccoli and leeks. Continue cooking until cheese melts. Remove from heat and beat eggs with salt, pepper and nutmeg. Add to broccoli mixture. Stir in almonds and turn into greased baking dish. Bake 40 min. at 350 degrees.

Serves 4.

SHRIMP CURRIED BROCCOLI

1 (10 oz.) pkg. frozen broccoli spears
1 cup Shrimp Curry Soup (p. 42)
3 Tbsp. Parmesan cheese, grated

Cook broccoli until barely tender. Place spears in shallow greased baking dish. Mix in Shrimp Curry Soup and top with cheese. Place in broiler until bubbly and lightly browned.

Serves 2–4.

COTTAGE-BROCCOLI SOUFFLÉ

3 eggs
Salt and pepper, to taste
1 pt. cottage cheese
1 (10 oz.) pkg. frozen chopped broccoli or ⅔ lb. fresh
½ cup sharp cheddar cheese, grated
3 Tbsp. butter

Beat eggs with salt and pepper. Combine with cottage cheese, broccoli and ¼ cup cheddar cheese. Melt butter in baking dish and turn broccoli mixture into it. Top with remaining ¼ cup cheddar cheese and bake 30 min. at 350 degrees.

Serves 6.

BROCCOLI SPECIALE

1 (10 oz.) pkg. frozen broccoli spears
3 Tbsp. butter
⅛ tsp. garlic powder
1½ tsp. Parmesan cheese, grated

Cook broccoli. Melt butter in small pan. Add garlic powder and grated Parmesan cheese. Mix well and pour over drained broccoli.

Suggestions:

This is especially good when zucchini is substituted for broccoli.

Try this butter sauce over asparagus, brussels sprouts or string beans. It can be used successfully with almost any vegetable.

Serves 4.

CAULIFLOWER AMANDINE

½ tsp. salt
1 (10 oz.) pkg. frozen cauliflower or ⅔ lb. fresh, cooked
1 clove garlic, minced
⅓ cup almonds, slivered
For Liberal Diet, add ½ cup Gluten Bread Crumbs, p. 143.
2½ Tbsp. butter

Sprinkle salt over cauliflower. Sauté garlic, almonds (and Crumbs) in butter. When slightly browned, spoon mixture over cauliflower and mix.

Serves 3–4.

GARLIC-CHEESE CAULIFLOWER

1 (10 oz.) pkg. frozen cauliflower
1 cup Garlic Cheese Sauce (p. 58)
Chives

Cook cauliflower in usual manner. Top with Garlic Cheese Sauce and sprinkle with chives.

Suggestions: This sauce is delicious over a variety of green vegetables.

Serves 3–4.

CREAMED CAULIFLOWER

1 (10 oz.) pkg. frozen cauliflower or
⅔ lb. fresh, cooked
1 Tbsp. parsley
¼ cup toasted almonds, slivered
¾ cup cheddar cheese, grated
1 cup White Cream Sauce, hot (p. 55)

Cut cauliflower into bite-size pieces. Combine with parsley and almonds. Sprinkle with cheese and top with White Cream Sauce.

Serves 4.

ASPARAGUS IN SOUR CREAM SAUCE

1 (10 oz.) pkg. frozen asparagus
1 cup Cream of Chicken Soup (p. 46)
½ cup sour cream
For Liberal Diet, add French Croutons, p. 145.

Cook asparagus until tender. Heat Cream of Chicken Soup and sour cream. (Toss in French Croutons.) Spoon over asparagus.

Serves 3–4.

ASPARAGUS FAN FARE

1 cup cottage cheese
1 cup sour cream
¼ tsp. salt
½ tsp. lemon juice
1 lb. asparagus, heated through
1 (4 oz.) can mushrooms, sliced and drained
¼ cup parsley, chopped

Combine cottage cheese and sour cream. Heat slowly, stirring constantly. Mix salt and lemon juice. Toss with asparagus. Add mushrooms and mix with melted cheese mixture. Turn into buttered casserole dish and top with parsley. Bake 25 min. at 325 degrees.

Serves 5–6.

MARINATED SHRIMP AND ARTICHOKE JUBILEE

2 (15 oz.) cans artichoke hearts, halved
1½ lb. (about 40) med. shrimp
½ cup vegetable oil
½ cup olive oil
½ cup wine vinegar
1 egg
2 Tbsp. Dijon-style mustard
2 Tbsp. chives, chopped
½ tsp. onion powder
½ tsp. salt
Sugar substitute equivalent to ½ tsp. sugar
Dash pepper

Chill artichokes and shrimp thoroughly. Combine all remaining ingredients in blender and process until smooth. Marinate artichokes and shrimp in mixture for at least 6 hrs.

Serves 6–8.

CABBAGE-MUSHROOM SUBLIME

2 cups mushrooms, sliced
2 cups bean sprouts
1 cup chives, chopped
2 Tbsp. oil
½ sm. head cabbage, shredded
Soy sauce, to taste

Sauté mushrooms, bean sprouts and chives in oil. Add cabbage and sprinkle with soy sauce. Cover and simmer 5 min.

Serves 4.

PUNGENT MARINATED MUSHROOMS

1 lb. sm. mushrooms
¼ cup water
½ cup oil
¾ cup red wine vinegar
1 tsp. tarragon
¼ tsp. salt
1 bay leaf, crumbled
¼ tsp. garlic powder
1 Tbsp. chives, chopped

Wipe mushrooms with damp towel. Combine remaining ingredients and pour over mushrooms. Refrigerate, covered, for 14 hrs., turning occasionally.

Suggestion: These are delicious in salads and very impressive as hors d'oeuvres.

Serves 6–8.

MUSHROOM NEWBURG

1½ lbs. med. mushrooms
¼ cup butter
3 Tbsp. chives, chopped
½ cup dry red wine
1½ cups White Cream Sauce, omitting cream of tartar (p. 55)
Dash cayenne
Dash nutmeg
2 egg yolks
2 Tbsp. cold water

Wipe mushrooms with damp towel. Melt butter in pan. Add mushrooms. Sauté until almost tender. Add chives and wine. Simmer 2 min. in White Cream Sauce, cayenne and nutmeg.

Beat egg yolks with water and add to mushroom mixture. Simmer for an additional 1 min.

Suggestion: For Liberal Diet, serve over Gluten Pasta.

Serves 4–6.

DELECTABLE FRENCH GREEN BEANS

½ cup water chestnuts
1 (10 oz.) pkg. frozen French-cut green beans, cooked
1 cup Cream of Mushroom Soup (p. 46)
For Liberal Diet, add Deep-Fried Onion Rings, p. 156.

Slice water chestnuts. Cook with green beans. Heat Cream of Mushroom Soup; then mix with vegetables. (Arrange Onion Rings on top and broil 1 min. to heat.)

Serves 4.

SWISS GREEN BEANS IN SOUR CREAM SAUCE

1½ Tbsp. butter
Sugar substitute equivalent to ½ tsp. sugar
½ tsp. onion powder
½ tsp. salt
½ cup sour cream
2 (10 oz.) pkgs. frozen green beans, heated through
1 cup Swiss cheese, grated

Melt butter in pan. Stir in sugar substitute, onion powder, salt and sour cream. Mix with beans and place in buttered baking pan. Cover with Swiss cheese. Bake at 350 degrees for about 20 min.

Serves 6.

GREEN BEAN BAKE

- ½ cup chives, chopped
- 3 Tbsp. butter
- 1 tsp. salt
- ¼ tsp. pepper
- 1 cup sour cream
- 2 cups green beans, cooked until almost tender
- ⅔ cups sharp cheddar cheese, grated

Sauté chives in butter and add salt, pepper and sour cream. Mix well and heat thoroughly. Combine with green beans and spoon into baking dish. Sprinkle cheese over top and broil until cheese melts.

Serves 3–4.

PETIT STRING BEAN SOUFFLÉS

- ¾ cup White Cream Sauce (p. 55)
- ¾ lb. string beans, cooked until tender
- 2 eggs, separated
- Dash onion powder
- Salt and pepper, as desired
- Butter
- ½ cup Cheese Sauce (p. 58)

Combine White Cream Sauce and ½ lb. string beans in blender. Process until smooth. Stir in beaten egg yolks, onion powder and remaining ¼ lb. string beans, diced. Salt and pepper as desired. Fold in egg whites beaten until stiff and moist. Butter custard cups and spoon in string bean mixture. Bake at 375 degrees for 20–25 min. or until knife inserted in center comes out clean. Pour hot Cheese Sauce over each soufflé before serving.

Variations:
Substitute peas for string beans.
Add chopped nuts to mixture before baking.

Serves 4–6.

BEAN SPROUT CASSEROLE

1 lb. bean sprouts
½ lb. water chestnuts
2½ cups Cream of Mushroom Soup (p. 46)
For Liberal Diet, add Buttered Gluten Crumbs, p. 143.

Heat bean sprouts with water chestnuts. Remove to casserole dish, pour Mushroom Soup over top. (Sprinkle with Crumbs.) Bake at 350 degrees until piping hot.

Serves 8.

ZUCCHINI BAKE

1 (10 oz.) pkg. frozen zucchini
¼ cup chives, chopped
⅓ cup green pepper, diced
Butter
2 tomatoes, diced
1 Tbsp. lemon juice
2 cloves garlic, minced
¼ tsp. salt
Dash pepper

Cook zucchini until almost tender. Sauté chives and green pepper in butter. Add remaining ingredients. Stir in zucchini and serve.

Suggestion: Spoon Zucchini Bake over salmon or halibut fillets.

Serves 3–4.

EGGPLANT IN CHEESE SAUCE

1 med. eggplant
2 Tbsp. butter
¼ tsp. salt
⅛ tsp. cayenne
1½ cups Cheese Sauce (p. 58)

Slice eggplant into ¼-in. thick slices. Sauté in butter 4–5 min. on first side. Turn and cook until golden brown. Sprinkle with salt. Add cayenne to Cheese Sauce and spoon over eggplant.

Serves 2–4.

ALMOND SPINACH

2 (10 oz.) pkgs. frozen spinach, chopped
1 cup Tomato-Cheese Sauce (p. 58)
½ cup almonds, slivered

Cook spinach. Heat Tomato-Cheese Sauce; then spoon over spinach. Top with almonds. Broil to toast almonds, if desired.

Serves 6.

SPINACH IN NUTMEG SAUCE

1 (10 oz.) pkg. frozen spinach
1 cup Nutmeg Sauce (p. 53)

Cook spinach in usual manner. Heat Nutmeg Sauce, then spoon over spinach. Serve immediately.

Suggestion: For Liberal Diet, serve this sauce over onions or carrots.

Serves 2–4.

SPINACH MARINARA

1 (10 oz.) pkg. frozen spinach
6 strips bacon, cooked and crumbled
2½–3 cups Marinara Sauce (p. 56)

Cook spinach. Mix with bacon bits. Heat Marinara Sauce, then spoon over spinach.

Serves 2–4.

CARAWAY-SPINACH BAKE

1 cup cottage cheese
1 tsp. salt
¼ tsp. pepper
Dash Worcestershire sauce
2 eggs
1 tsp. caraway seeds
½ tsp. celery seeds
2 Tbsp. walnuts, chopped
1 (10 oz.) pkg. frozen spinach, chopped
½ cup sharp cheddar cheese, grated

Combine cottage cheese, salt, pepper and Worcestershire sauce in blender and mix until smooth. Add eggs, caraway and celery seeds. Process quickly to blend. Add walnuts. Combine mixture with spinach and turn into greased baking dish. Sprinkle cheese over top and bake 20 min. at 350 degrees.

Serves 4.

Entrees

BEEF CHOW MEIN

2 lbs. round steak, trimmed and cut into ¼ x 2-in. strips
Salt and pepper
Butter
⅔ cup soy sauce
⅔ cup dry white wine
½ tsp. ginger
1½ cups water
2 cups green peppers, diced
1½ cups water chestnuts, sliced
4 cups bean sprouts
2 cups celery, diced
1¾ cups chives, chopped
For Liberal Diet, substitute 1¾ cups diced onion.
1 tsp. Teriyaki sauce

Season meat with salt and pepper. Brown well in butter. Add soy sauce, wine, ginger and water. Cover and simmer until meat is tender, about 2 hrs. Sauté green peppers, water chestnuts, bean sprouts, celery and chives in a small amount of butter. Cover and simmer vegetables for 10–15 min. or until soft. Add vegetables and liquid to meat. Add Teriyaki sauce; cover and simmer 5–10 min.

Variations:

Substitute pork for beef to make PORK CHOW MEIN.
Substitute chicken for beef to make CHICKEN CHOW MEIN.
Substitute shrimp for beef to make SHRIMP CHOW MEIN.
For Liberal Diet, serve over Mock Gluten Rice.

Serves 6–8.

BEEF JERKY

1 ½-lb. flank steak (beef)
⅓ cup soy sauce
1 tsp. garlic powder
1 tsp. dehydrated parsley flakes
¼ tsp. onion powder
Dash salt and pepper

Trim meat and cut into ¼-in. wide strips, with the grain. Marinate 4 hrs. in mixture of soy sauce, garlic powder, parsley flakes, onion powder, salt and pepper. Arrange strips on rack placed on baking sheet. Bake 5–6 hrs. at 150 degrees. Remove from oven and cool. Use for snacks.

TERRY'S STEAK KABOBS

1¼ lbs. top sirloin, cubed
Teriyaki sauce, to cover
Garlic, to taste
2 Tbsp. butter
1 clove garlic, pressed
For Liberal Diet, add 1 lg. onion, cut into small wedges.
½ lb. whole mushrooms
1 lg. green pepper, cut into small pieces

Marinate cubed meat in Teriyaki sauce and garlic for at least 6 hrs. Melt butter in pan and add 1 clove garlic. Sauté (onion and) mushrooms. Add 2 Tbsp. marinade to mixture in pan. Stir well and add green pepper and drained meat. String meat and vegetables onto skewers. Barbecue or broil until done as desired, about 3 min.

Variation: For Liberal Diet, sauté green pepper with onions and mushrooms. Broil meat, then add to pan mixture. Serve over Gluten Egg Noodles.

Serves 4.

HAMBURGER STEAK PRODIGY

1½ lbs. ground beef
1 egg
For Liberal Diet, add ½ cup Gluten Bread Crumbs, *p. 143.*
Salt and pepper, as desired
½ tsp. M.S.G. (monosodium glutamate)
¼ tsp. garlic powder
¾ tsp. onion powder
1½ cups Cheese Sauce (p. 58)

Mix ground beef with egg, (Crumbs), salt, pepper, M.S.G., garlic powder and onion powder. Form into 4 steaks. Fry or broil as desired. Top with hot Cheese Sauce and serve immediately.

Variations:

Top with Swiss Cheese Sauce.
Top with Cream of Mushroom Soup.
Bake with Italian Spaghetti Sauce.

Serves 4.

LASAGNA

4½ cups Italian Spaghetti Sauce, warm (p. 57)
2 zucchini, sliced thin lengthwise
For Liberal Diet, substitute double recipe Gluten Pasta, cut into wide Lasagna Noodles, *p. 142.*
16 oz. ricotta cheese
½ cup Parmesan cheese, grated
8 oz. mozzarella cheese, sliced

Using slotted spoon, cover bottom of baking dish with spaghetti sauce. Place zucchini slices in layer over sauce. Layer ricotta over zucchini and sprinkle with Parmesan cheese. Spoon sauce generously over cheese, followed by half the mozzarella, zucchini, ricotta, Parmesan, sauce, zucchini and remaining mozzarella cheese. Bake at 375 degrees for 30–35 min.

Serves 4.

LASAGNA CASSEROLE

Meat Mixture:

1 lb. ground beef
¼ tsp. garlic powder
1 Tbsp. parsley flakes
¼ tsp. salt
½ tsp. oregano
½ tsp. basil
⅛ tsp. pepper
Onion powder, to taste
¾ cup tomato paste

Cheese Mixture:

1 egg
⅓ cup Parmesan cheese, grated
1 cup small curd cottage cheese
4 oz. mozzarella cheese, sliced

Cook ground beef until light brown, drain and add remaining meat mixture ingredients. Simmer until hot. Combine ingredients for cheese mixture and set aside. Spoon half of meat mixture into casserole dish. Cover evenly with cheese mixture. Layer remaining meat mixture over cheese layer and top with mozzarella cheese slices. Bake at 350 degrees until cheese melts and sauce is bubbling hot.

Serves 4.

MING MUSHROOM ROAST BEEF

1 lb. mushrooms
⅓ cup butter
1 Tbsp. chives, chopped
Brown sugar substitute equivalent to 1 tsp. sugar
1 tsp. soy sauce
½ cup chicken broth
For Liberal Diet, add 1 tsp. gluten flour.
6 slices cooked roast beef

Remove ends of stems and slice mushrooms. Sauté in butter until almost tender. Combine remaining ingredients and add to mushrooms. Continue cooking over low heat until tender. Spoon over hot roast beef slices.

Serves 4.

COTTAGE MEATBALLS

1 lb. ground beef
1 egg
For Liberal Diet, add ½ cup Gluten Bread Crumbs, p. 143.
½ tsp. salt
¼ tsp. pepper
½ tsp. nutmeg
⅔ cup water
1 pt. cottage cheese, drained and rinsed
Sugar substitute equivalent to 3 tsp. sugar
1 tsp. dehydrated parsley flakes
1 Tbsp. oil

Combine meat with egg, (Crumbs), salt, pepper and nutmeg. Shape into balls. In blender, mix water, cottage cheese, sugar substitute and parsley flakes. Process until smooth. Heat oil in pan and brown meatballs on all sides. Cover and simmer until almost done, about 10 min. Drain. Pour sauce over meatballs and heat, stirring occasionally.

Note: Too much handling tends to make any meatballs hard.

Suggestion: For Liberal Diet, increase amount of sauce and serve over Gluten Egg Noodles.

Serves 4.

SPICY MEATBALLS IN TOMATO SAUCE

1 lb. ground beef
1 egg, slightly beaten
½ tsp. salt
⅛ tsp. pepper
¼ cup Basic Tomato Sauce (p. 61)
¼ tsp. paprika
¼ tsp. Worcestershire sauce
For Liberal Diet, add ½ cup Gluten Bread Crumbs, p. 143.
2 Tbsp. chives, chopped
1 Tbsp. oil
2 cups Basic Tomato Sauce (p. 61)
1½ cups beef bouillon
2 Tbsp. lemon juice
Sugar substitute equivalent to 2 tsp. sugar
½ tsp. basil leaves
Dash M.S.G. (monosodium glutamate)

Mix meat with egg, salt, pepper, ¼ cup Basic Tomato Sauce, paprika, Worcestershire, (Crumbs) and chives. Form into balls. Drop them into hot oil and brown on all sides. Cover and cook until nearly done. Pour off fat and combine 2 cups Basic Tomato Sauce, bouillon, lemon juice, sugar substitute, basil leaves and M.S.G. Add sauce to meatball pan and simmer until sauce is hot and meatballs are done.

Serves 4.

MEATBALLS MARINARA

1 lb. ground beef
2 Tbsp. parsley, chopped fine
For Liberal Diet, add ½ cup Gluten Bread Crumbs, p. 143.
2 cloves garlic, minced
2 Tbsp. Parmesan cheese, grated
⅛ tsp. onion powder
¼ tsp. pepper
1 egg, slightly beaten
Oil, for cooking
2½–3 cups Marinara Sauce (p. 56)

Combine meat with all ingredients except Marinara Sauce. Form into balls and brown on all sides in oil. Cover and simmer until done as desired, about 15 min. Drain, spoon Marinara Sauce over meatballs and serve.

Suggestion: For Liberal Diet, serve over Gluten Egg Noodles.

Serves 4.

MEATBALLS IN SOUR CREAM

1 lb. ground beef
For Liberal Diet, add ½ cup Gluten Bread Crumbs, p. 143.
½ tsp. salt
¼ tsp. onion powder
½ tsp. nutmeg
1 egg, slightly beaten
1 Tbsp. oil
1 pt. sour cream
2 Tbsp. parsley, chopped

Combine beef with (Crumbs), salt, onion powder, nutmeg and egg. Brown on all sides in oil, cover and cook until nearly done, 10–15 min. Remove to baking dish. Mix sour cream with parsley and spoon over meatballs. Bake at 350 degrees for 10 min. or until sour cream is hot.

Variations:

Omit parsley and add brussels sprouts to cream.

For Liberal Diet, omit parsley and add peas to sour cream.

Serves 4.

MEATBALL SURPRISE WITH VEGETABLES

- 1 lb. ground beef
- ½ tsp. salt
- ¼ tsp. pepper
- ¼ tsp. garlic powder
- ⅛ tsp. onion powder
  For Liberal Diet, add ¼ cup Gluten Bread Crumbs, p. 143.
- 1 egg, slightly beaten
- 3 oz. sharp cheddar cheese, cut into ¼-in. cubes
- ½ lb. mushroom caps
- ½ lb. cherry tomatoes
- 1½ cups green peppers, diced
- 4 cups beef bouillon

Season ground beef with salt, pepper, garlic powder and onion powder. Combine with (Crumbs and) egg. Shape into balls around cheese cubes. Drop vegetables into boiling bouillon for 2 min. Add meatballs and cook for an additional 3 min. Spoon out meat and vegetables onto serving platter.

Serves 4–6.

FLANK STEAK ORIENTAL

1 lb. flank steak
⅓ cup soy sauce
4 tsp. chives, chopped
For Liberal Diet, substitute 4 tsp. minced onion and omit onion powder.
1 tsp. garlic powder
1 tsp. dehydrated parsley flakes
Dash salt
Dash pepper
¼ tsp. onion powder

Marinate steak in mixture of remaining ingredients for at least 2 hrs. Broil 10–15 min. each side or until meat is browned and done as preferred. Slice at an extreme angle in thin strips. Spoon any remaining marinade over sliced steak and serve immediately. (Meat cools very rapidly.)

Suggestion: Substitute pork chops for flank steak and barbecue.

Serves 4.

STEAK DIANE SUPERB

2 Tbsp. shallots, sliced
5 Tbsp. butter
4 sirloin steaks, trimmed and pounded thin
2 Tbsp. chives, chopped
2 Tbsp. parsley, chopped fine
Dash Worcestershire sauce
Dash steak sauce
Dash salt and pepper, or to taste

Sauté shallots in butter until golden brown. Add steaks and sear on both sides. Add chives, parsley, Worcestershire sauce and steak sauce. Stir mixture and continue to cook until steaks are as desired. Season with salt and pepper, and serve.

Serves 4.

BROCHETTE OF BEEF

⅓ cup dry white wine
1 cup soy sauce
2 tsp. garlic powder
¼ tsp. ginger
Sugar substitute equivalent to 3 tsp. sugar
1 lb. beef tenderloin, trimmed and cut into cubes
Mushroom caps
Cherry tomatoes
Green peppers, cut into squares
For Liberal Diet, add onion wedges.

Mix wine, soy sauce, garlic powder, ginger and sugar substitute. Marinate beef for several hours. Drain and alternate meat and vegetables on skewers. Broil, basting occasionally with marinade, until meat is done as desired.

Note: Especially good when mushrooms, (onions) and peppers are sautéed in butter to soften before broiling.

Serves 6.

MEXICAN MEAT LOAF

1 lb. lean ground beef
Salt and pepper, as desired
1 egg, slightly beaten
⅛ tsp. garlic powder
1 Tbsp. ketchup
⅛ tsp. cayenne
For Liberal Diet, add ⅓ cup Oven-Dried Gluten Bread Crumbs, p. 143.

Mix meat with remaining ingredients in a bowl. Form loaf and place in a baking dish. Bake at 425 degrees for 10 min. or until loaf is slightly browned and fat has melted. Pour off fat and return to 350 degree oven for 40 min. or until done as desired. Slice and serve.

Serves 4.

BEEF STROGANOFF

1½ lbs. top round steak, trimmed and cut into julienne strips, 2 x ¼-in.
Salt and pepper, as desired
Dash garlic powder
2 Tbsp. butter
1 cup dry white wine
2 cups water
⅛ cup dry white wine
1 pt. sour cream

Season meat with salt, pepper and garlic powder. Melt butter in frying pan and add meat. Brown, reduce heat and add 1 cup wine and water. Simmer, covered, until meat is tender, about 2 hrs.

Meanwhile, prepare Stroganoff Sauce as follows:

1 oz. mushrooms
Dash onion powder
Dash cream of tartar
Dash M.S.G. (monosodium glutamate)
Dash pepper
⅛ tsp. salt
½ tsp. celery, diced
¼ tsp. dehydrated parsley flakes
1 Tbsp. butter
Sugar substitute equivalent to ¼ tsp. sugar
½ cup heavy cream
For Liberal Diet, substitute ½ cup light cream.
3 water chestnuts
For Liberal Diet, substitute 1 slice gluten bread.

Combine all ingredients in a blender until smooth. When meat is tender, pour off pan liquid into a container. Return ⅛ cup liquid to pan and add ⅛ cup wine. Add ⅔ cup Stroganoff Sauce and simmer, covered, for 5 min. Add sour cream and heat but do not allow to boil.

Suggestion: For Liberal Diet, serve over Gluten Egg Noodles or Mock Gluten Rice.

Serves 4.

CREAMED FRANKS DIVINE

1½ cups sour cream
⅓ cup ketchup
⅓ cup prepared mustard
Garlic salt, to taste
10 frankfurters, cooked

Combine sour cream, ketchup, mustard and garlic salt. Heat and spoon over hot franks.

Suggestion: Cocktail frankfurters in this sauce make tasty hors d'oeuvres.

Serves 5.

GRENADINE OF BEEF

½ lb. mushrooms
⅔ cup chives, chopped
For Liberal Diet, substitute ⅔ cups scallions.
⅛ lb. butter
Pinch each: oregano, basil, marjoram
4 cloves garlic, minced
¾ cup dry red wine
11 oz. Cream of Mushroom Soup (p. 46)
1½ lbs. filet mignon steaks

Sauté mushrooms and chives in butter. Add oregano, basil, marjoram and garlic. Add wine and simmer 5–7 min. Add Cream of Mushroom Soup and simmer. Brown meat quickly in hot pan. Pour sauce over meat and serve.

Serves 2–4.

DELUXE PATTY MELTS

1½ lbs. ground beef
1 egg
For Liberal Diet, add ½ cup Gluten Bread Crumbs, p. 143.
½ tsp. salt
¼ tsp. pepper
¼ tsp. M.S.G. (monosodium glutamate)
4 slices tomato
4 slices Monterey Jack or other mild cheese
2 cups Avocado Sauce (p. 59)

Mix beef with egg, (Crumbs), salt, pepper and M.S.G. Form into 4 patties. Broil, turn and top each with a slice of tomato. Place a slice of cheese over tomato and complete cooking. Place each patty on a plate and cover with Avocado Sauce. (For Liberal Diet, serve over slices of gluten toast.)

Serves 4.

BEEF-STUFFED BELL PEPPERS

6 well-shaped bell peppers
½ cup chives, chopped
For Liberal Diet, substitute ½ cup chopped onion.
⅓ cup celery, diced
2 Tbsp. butter
1 lb. ground beef
⅛ tsp. pepper
¼ tsp. garlic powder
2 cups Basic Tomato Sauce (p. 61)
For Liberal Diet, add about 12 extra-sm. Croutons Parmesan, p. 144.
1 tsp. dehydrated parsley flakes
2 tsp. bell pepper, diced from removed tops
⅛ cup Oven-Dried Gluten Bread Crumbs (p. 143), optional

Slice tops off of bell peppers, clean and drain upside down. Sauté chives and celery in butter. Season meat with pepper and garlic powder. Add meat to vegetables and brown. Drain, add Basic Tomato Sauce, (Croutons), parsley flakes and bell pepper pieces. Cook over medium heat for 5 min. Spoon meat mixture into peppers and sprinkle with Crumbs. Place in pan and bake at 425 degrees for 15 min. Lower heat to 350 degrees and bake until peppers are soft.

Serves 6.

GREEN PEPPER SOY STEAK

2 lbs. skirt steak, trimmed and cut into ¼ x 2-in. strips
Salt and pepper, as desired
2 Tbsp. butter
⅔ cup soy sauce
⅔ cup dry white wine
½ tsp. ginger
1½ cups water
2 cups green pepper, diced
2 cups celery, diced
1½ cups chives, diced
For Liberal Diet, substitute 1½ cups onion.
1 tsp. Teriyaki sauce

Season meat with salt and pepper and brown in small amount of butter or oil. Pour off excess and add soy sauce, wine, ginger and water. Cover and simmer until meat is tender. Sauté green peppers, celery and chives in butter until soft. Add water to cover vegetables. Simmer 10 min., covered. Add vegetables and liquid to meat pan. Stir in Teriyaki sauce. Cover and simmer 5 min. Spoon onto plates.

Suggestion: For Liberal Diet, serve over Gluten Egg Noodles.

Serves 6.

SOY STYLE GROUND PORK

1 lb. ground pork
1 egg
For Liberal Diet, add ½ cup Oven-Dried Gluten Bread Crumbs, p. 143.
1 tsp. soy sauce
½ tsp. salt
1 tsp. onion powder
Oil
⅓ Tbsp. chives, chopped
1 tsp. dehydrated parsley flakes
1 tsp. garlic powder
Dash salt
Dash pepper

Mix pork with egg, (Crumbs), soy sauce, ½ tsp. salt and onion powder. Form into small balls. Brown on all sides in oil. Drain. Combine all remaining ingredients. Heat slowly and serve over cooked pork balls.

Variations:

Use soy sauce mixture as a marinade for pork loin roast.
Top pork chops with soy sauce mixture.

Serves 4.

TUNA BAKE PARMESAN

⅔ cup mayonnaise
1 Tbsp. ketchup
2 Tbsp. chili sauce
1 tsp. tarragon vinegar
½ tsp. paprika
½ tsp. celery salt
¼ tsp. dry mustard
2 (7 oz.) cans tuna, drained and chunked
Parmesan cheese, grated

Combine all ingredients except cheese. Turn into baking pan and sprinkle cheese generously over top. Bake at 350 degrees for 15 min. or until cheese melts and mixture is hot.

Serves 4.

SALMON LOAF SUPREME

Loaf:

2 (1 lb.) cans red salmon
1 Tbsp. dehydrated parsley flakes or 6–8 sprigs fresh, chopped fine
¼ tsp. salt
2 Tbsp. chives, chopped fine
For Liberal Diet, add 2 Tbsp. Buttered Gluten Crumbs, p. 143.
5 oz. mayonnaise
1 tsp. sesame seeds
1 tsp. celery seeds
2 Tbsp. butter, melted

Drain and clean salmon. Flake well and combine with parsley, salt, chives, (Crumbs) and mayonnaise. Form into a loaf and place in baking dish. Bake at 400 degrees for 15 min. Sprinkle with seeds, drizzle with butter and bake for an additional 10 min.

Sauce:

1 (1 lb.) can whole tomatoes
Sugar substitute equivalent to 1 tsp. sugar
¾ cup celery, diced
½ cup bell pepper, diced
½ cup heavy cream
Dash salt and pepper

Spoon tomatoes into blender. Process at medium speed until liquefied thoroughly. Add sugar substitute to 1 cup of the purée, pour into saucepan and add celery, bell pepper, cream, salt and pepper. Simmer 15 min. while loaf is baking. Garnish loaf with romaine and parsley sprigs. Serve sauce spooned over individual servings.

Serves 4.

SALMON CROQUETTES

1 (1 lb.) can salmon, drained and cleaned
For Liberal Diet, add 1/8 cup Gluten Bread Crumbs, p. 143.
1 Tbsp. lemon juice
1 Tbsp. light cream
2 Tbsp. parsley, chopped fine
2 Tbsp. chives, chopped fine
1½ Tbsp. celery, chopped fine
Dash pepper
2 Tbsp. butter
For Liberal Diet, add raw onion rings.

Flake salmon into bowl. Add other ingredients, except butter, and mix well. Form into patties and fry in butter. (Place raw onion rings in pan around patties, if desired.) Turn croquettes after cooking 5 min. over medium heat. Fry for an additional 5 min. and serve (with onion rings on top of croquettes, if used).

Variations:

Patties may be broiled instead of fried. Dot with butter.
Pour Cream of Tomato Soup over croquettes.
Serve topped with Cream of Mushroom Soup.

Makes 4–5.

TERIYAKI SALMON STEAKS

½ cup Teriyaki sauce
½ tsp. garlic powder
1 tsp. lemon juice
4 salmon steaks

Combine Teriyaki sauce, garlic and lemon juice. Use as a marinade for the salmon. Allow to stand 3–5 hrs. Broil until done as desired.

Serves 4.

MOCK SALMON CASSEROLE

½ cup green pepper, diced
¾ cup celery, diced
2 cups Basic Tomato Sauce (p. 61)
2 cups heavy cream
2 (13 oz.) cans albacore tuna

In a saucepan, combine green peppers, celery and Basic Tomato Sauce. Simmer 15 min. or until vegetables soften. Add cream and stir. Mix in tuna and heat thoroughly.

Variations for Liberal Diet:

Prepare tuna and sauce. Pour over Stretch-Cut Gluten Toast. This makes a tasty and easily prepared quick snack or lunch.

Serve over Gluten Egg Noodles.

Serves 4–6.

KING CRAB BROCCOLI WITH CHEESE SAUCE

2 (10 oz.) pkgs. frozen broccoli spears, cooked until almost tender
2 (7¾ oz.) cans king crab meat
2 cups Cheese Sauce (p. 58)
1 (4 oz.) can sliced mushrooms, drained
¼ cup dry red wine
¼ cup Parmesan cheese, grated

Layer broccoli into buttered casserole dish. Remove membrane from crab meat and reserve 6 lg. pieces. Flake remaining crab meat and combine with Cheese Sauce, mushrooms and wine. Arrange reserved crab meat over broccoli and top with Cheese Sauce mixture. Sprinkle with Parmesan cheese and bake 15 min. at 400 degrees.

Serves 4–6.

JACK CHEESE TURBOT

1 cup Monterey Jack or other mild cheese, grated
1½ tsp. dehydrated parsley flakes
1 lg. piece turbot, cut into 4 pieces
Butter
Lemon juice

Combine cheese and parsley flakes in bowl. Broil turbot with butter and lemon juice. Turn fish over and top with cheese mixture last 3 min. of cooking time.

Serves 4.

STUFFED LOBSTER BRANDY

¼ cup butter, melted
2 cups heavy cream
1 tsp. salt
Dash pepper
Dash onion powder
1 tsp. dry mustard
½ cup dry red wine
12 water chestnuts
For Liberal Diet, substitute 2 slices gluten bread.
½–¾ tsp. imitation brandy flavoring
½ cup mushrooms, sliced and sautéed
2 cooked lobsters, split and diced
¼ cup mozzarella cheese, grated

Combine butter, cream, salt, pepper, onion powder, mustard and wine in blender container. With blender running, add 2 water chestnuts at a time until desired consistency is achieved. Pour into saucepan and add brandy flavoring. Cook, stirring constantly, until mixture is hot. Add mushrooms and lobster to sauce and heat. Fill lobster shells with mixture and top with cheese. Broil until cheese melts.

Serves 4.

BOILED LIVE MAINE LOBSTER

4 lobsters
Water to cover
1 Tbsp. salt per qt. water
Melted butter
Lemon wedges

Place enough water in deep pot to cover lobsters. Add salt and bring to a boil. Place lobsters in water head first. Cover and simmer 9–10 min. Remove lobsters from water, drain and dry. Split lengthwise, crack claws, remove stomach, intestinal vein, roe and liver. (If desired, roe and liver may be retained.) Serve with butter and lemon.

Serves 4.

SHRIMP CREOLE

1 (1 lb., 12 oz.) can whole tomatoes
⅓ cup liquid from canned tomatoes
½ cup tomato paste
¼ tsp. onion powder
1 tsp. parsley flakes
Dash Tabasco sauce
¼ tsp. salt
1½ cups green pepper, diced
1 cup celery, diced
2 Tbsp. butter
2 lbs. shrimp
½ cup dry white wine
1 bay leaf

Combine tomatoes, liquid, tomato paste, onion powder, parsley flakes, Tabasco and salt in blender. Process until smooth. Sauté green pepper and celery in butter until tender. Add to sauce. Pour into saucepan and add shrimp and wine. Place bay leaf on top and simmer for 20 min. Remove bay leaf and serve.

Serves 6.

SHRIMP IN WINE SAUCE

½ cup butter
2 Tbsp. parsley, chopped
1 Tbsp. lemon juice
¼ tsp. salt
½ cup dry white wine
¼ tsp. garlic powder
½ tsp. prepared mustard
Dash thyme
2 doz. lg. raw shrimp, deveined and in shells (Snip with scissors to devein.)

Melt butter in pan and add parsley, lemon juice, salt, wine, garlic powder, mustard and thyme. Cook over low heat for 4–5 min. Stand shrimp in shallow pan and brush with hot mixture, reserving some for serving on top. Broil for 5 min.

Serves 4.

OYSTER-SHRIMP TARRAGON

1 lb. shrimp, deveined and shelled
½ cup chives, chopped
For Liberal Diet, substitute ½ cup scallions.
2 Tbsp. butter
1 lb. oysters, shelled
2 Tbsp. lemon juice
Generous ½ tsp. tarragon
Dash garlic powder
½ cup dry white wine
2 Tbsp. parsley, chopped fine

Cut shrimp lengthwise. Sauté chives in butter. Add shrimp, oysters, lemon juice, tarragon and garlic powder. Stir over high heat until shrimp and oysters are soft, 5–6 min. Put mixture in baking dish, adding wine and parsley. Broil for 5 min.

Serves 4–6.

SHRIMP IN TOMATO SAUCE

1 cup chives, chopped
For Liberal Diet, substitute 1 cup onion.
¾ cup celery, diced
¾ cup green pepper, diced
2 Tbsp. butter
½ cup dry white wine
1½ cups Basic Tomato Sauce (p. 61)
2 lbs. shrimp, cleaned and cooked
¼ tsp. garlic powder
¼ tsp. thyme
¼ tsp. basil
Salt and pepper, as desired
Parsley, chopped

Sauté chives, celery and pepper in butter until soft. Stir in wine and Basic Tomato Sauce. Add shrimp, garlic powder, thyme, basil, salt and pepper. Simmer 10 min. Sprinkle parsley over top and serve.

Serves 4–6.

MUSSEL DELIGHT

3 qts. mussels, scrubbed
½ cup chives, chopped
¼ cup dehydrated parsley flakes
¼ tsp. thyme
½ tsp. celery seeds
¼ tsp. basil
1 Tbsp. butter
Salt and pepper, as desired

Place rinsed mussels in large saucepan and add all remaining ingredients. Cover and cook over medium heat 10–12 min. Remove any unopened mussels and shells. Serve using pan mixture over top of mussels.

Serves 4.

CRAB IN SOUR CREAM SAUCE

1 lb. crab meat, flaked
⅓ cup sour cream
¾ cup mayonnaise
1 cup green pepper, chopped
¾ cup celery, chopped
1 Tbsp. Dijon mustard
2 Tbsp. lemon juice
2 hard-boiled eggs, chopped
For Liberal Diet, add ½ cup Buttered Gluten Crumbs, p. 143.
⅓ cup Romano cheese, grated

Mix crab with sour cream, mayonnaise, green pepper, celery, mustard, lemon juice and eggs. Place in buttered baking dish and top with (Crumbs and) Romano cheese. Bake at 350 degrees for 15–18 min.

Serves 4.

SHRIMP IN AVOCADO SAUCE

2 lbs. shrimp, deveined and shelled
3 Tbsp. butter
1 (1 lb.) can whole tomatoes, drained
2 cups Avocado Sauce (p. 59)
Salt and pepper, to taste
1 Tbsp. dehydrated parsley flakes
For Liberal Diet, add Gluten Egg Noodles, p. 142.

Cook shrimp in butter 5–8 min. or until soft. Mash tomatoes into Avocado Sauce. Pour sauce into shrimp pan and stir while heating slowly. Remove from heat. Salt and pepper, to taste. Serve sprinkled with parsley.

Suggestion: For Liberal Diet, spoon over Gluten Egg Noodles.

Serves 4–6.

SAND DABS IN CREAM SAUCE

4 Tbsp. butter
2 lbs. sand dabs
2 Tbsp. lemon juice
1 cup White Cream Sauce (p. 55)
2 Tbsp. parsley, chopped

Melt butter in pan. Add sand dabs and sprinkle with lemon juice. Fry, uncovered, until fish is flaky and white. Remove to serving plates and pour White Cream Sauce over the top. Sprinkle with parsley.

Serves 4.

SCALLOPS WITH A FOREIGN FLAIR

4 Tbsp. butter
½ tsp. garlic powder
Dash onion powder
2 lbs. scallops
½ lb. mushrooms, sliced
½ cup water chestnuts, sliced
1 cup bean sprouts
½ cup chives, chopped
1 Tbsp. soy sauce
½ cup dry white wine

Melt butter in pan. Add garlic and onion powder. Sauté scallops 5 min., or until partially cooked. Add mushrooms, water chestnuts, bean sprouts and chives. Cook until vegetables are tender. Add soy sauce and wine. Heat thoroughly.

Variations:
Substitute shrimp for scallops.
Add a favorite vegetable.

Serves 6.

TROUT WITH MARINATED MUSHROOMS

4 trout
2 Tbsp. lemon juice
3 Tbsp. butter, melted
½ tsp. salt
Pungent Marinated Mushrooms (p. 72)

Place trout on broiling pan and sprinkle generously with lemon juice. Cover with butter. Broil 7–8 min. on each side, topping with Mushrooms last 2 min. of cooking time.

Serves 4.

CREAMED OYSTERS

¼ tsp. onion powder
1 cup, half light cream, half water
For Liberal Diet, substitute 1 cup milk.
1 cup heavy cream
1 Tbsp. Worcestershire sauce
1 Tbsp. butter
1 (8 oz.) can whole oysters, with liquid
2 Tbsp. parsley, chopped
1 tsp. paprika
1 tsp. fennel seeds, optional
Salt and pepper, to taste

Combine all ingredients in saucepan and simmer until heated thoroughly. Do not boil.

Suggestions:
Combine oysters and clams for delicious stew.
For Liberal Diet, serve over Gluten Egg Noodles.

Serves 4.

SPICY CHEESE SCALLOPS

2 lbs. scallops
½ cup dry white wine
1 cup water
2 cups Garlic Cheese Sauce (p. 58)
2 Tbsp. chives, chopped

Simmer scallops in wine and water, covered, for 4–5 min. or until scallops are white and firm. Drain. Cover with Garlic Cheese Sauce and top with chives.

Serves 4–6.

CHICKEN MILANO

½ cup sunflower kernels
For Liberal Diet, substitute ½ cup Oven-Dried Gluten Bread Crumbs, p. 143.
¼ cup Parmesan cheese, grated
½ tsp. salt
¼ tsp. pepper
1 broiler-fryer, cut up, *or*
4 whole chicken breasts, boned, skinned and split
1 egg, slightly beaten
Equal amounts of oil and butter, as needed

Crush sunflower kernels in blender until they are the texture of fine bread crumbs. Combine with cheese, salt and pepper in paper bag. Rinse chicken pieces, drain and pat dry. Dip each in egg, then shake in nut mixture. Heat butter and oil in frying pan and add chicken to brown on both sides. Reduce heat and cover. Cook over low heat for 20–30 min. or until largest pieces are tender. Turn once to brown evenly and complete last 10 min. of cooking time uncovered.

Variation: Use Romano cheese in place of Parmesan.

Serves 4–6.

CHICKEN MILANO SUPREME

Chicken, coated with Crumb-Cheese mixture as for Chicken Milano (p. 103)
Equal amounts butter and oil, as needed
2 cups Italian Spaghetti Sauce (p. 57)
Swiss cheese, grated

Brown chicken in butter and oil on both sides. Drain chicken and add to sauce. Cover and simmer as for Chicken Milano. Sprinkle with Swiss cheese before serving.

Serves 4–6.

POPPY SEED CHICKEN

½ cup sesame seeds
For Liberal Diet, substitute ½ cup Oven-Dried Gluten Bread Crumbs, p. 143.
1 tsp. poppy seeds
For Liberal Diet, add 1½ Tbsp. sesame seeds.
1 tsp. salt
½ tsp. pepper
1 egg
1 Tbsp. light cream
1 broiler-fryer, cut up, *or*
3 whole chicken breasts, boned, skinned and split
Melted butter

Crush sesame seeds in blender until they are the texture of fine bread crumbs. Add poppy seeds, salt and pepper. Beat egg with cream. Dip chicken into egg mixture, then bread with seed mixture. Arrange in buttered baking dish and bake at 350 degrees for 30 min. Drizzle with melted butter and return to oven for an additional 25 min. or until done.

Variation: Top with hot Ginger Sauce just before serving.

Serves 4–6.

CHICKEN STROGANOFF

- ½ cup sunflower kernels
  For Liberal Diet, substitute ½ cup Gluten Bread Crumbs, p. 143.
- Dash salt and pepper
- 2 whole chicken breasts, boned, skinned, pounded thin and cut into 2 x ¼-in. strips
- 1 egg, beaten with 1 Tbsp. sour cream
- Equal amounts butter and oil, as needed
- 2 oz. mushrooms
- ¼ tsp. onion powder
- ¼ tsp. salt
- ⅛ tsp. pepper
- ¾ cup light cream
- 10–12 water chestnuts
  For Liberal Diet, substitute 2 slices gluten bread.
- 1 Tbsp. paprika
- ¼ cup dry white wine
- 1 tsp. Worcestershire sauce
- ¼ tsp. dehydrated parsley flakes
- 2 cups sour cream
- 3 cups bean sprouts, sautéed in butter
  For Liberal Diet, substitute Gluten Egg Noodles, p. 142.

Crush sunflower kernels in blender until they are the texture of fine bread crumbs. Combine with dash salt and pepper in a paper bag. Dip chicken strips in egg mixture, then shake in bag to coat. Brown chicken on both sides in butter and oil. In blender container, combine mushrooms, onion powder, salt, pepper, cream, water chestnuts, paprika, wine, Worcestershire sauce and parsley flakes. Blend until smooth. Heat mixture and add sour cream. Arrange chicken strips on bean sprouts and spoon sauce on top.

Serves 4–6.

CHEDDAR CHICKEN

3 whole chicken breasts, boned, skinned and split
Salt and pepper, as desired
Equal amounts butter and oil, as needed
1½ cups Cheese Sauce (p. 58)
⅓ cup dry white wine
½ tsp. rosemary

Season chicken with salt and pepper. Heat butter and oil in frying pan and add chicken. Cook 20 min. on each side, or until tender. Mix Cheese Sauce with wine and rosemary. Heat and spoon over chicken.

Serves 4–6.

FENNEL SEED CHICKEN

½ cup sesame seeds
For Liberal Diet, substitute ¼ cup Oven-Dried Gluten Bread Crumbs, p. 143.
1¼ tsp. fennel seeds
For Liberal Diet, add 4 tsp. sesame seeds.
1 tsp. salt
¼ tsp. pepper
3 whole chicken breasts, boned, skinned, split and pounded thin, *or*
1 broiler-fryer, cut up
1 egg
1 Tbsp. light cream
Equal amounts butter and oil, as needed

Crush sesame seeds in blender until they are the texture of fine bread crumbs. Add fennel seeds, (sesame seeds), salt and pepper. Beat egg with cream. Dip chicken in egg mixture, then bread with seed mixture. Set aside on wax paper for 10 min. Heat butter and oil in frying pan and add chicken. When chicken is golden brown, remove to buttered baking dish and bake, covered, at 350 degrees for 40 min. or until tender.

Variations:

Spoon Ginger Sauce over chicken.

Instead of frying chicken, bake 1 hr. at 350 degrees as an alternate method of cooking.

Serves 4–6.

CREAMED CHICKEN IN WINE SAUCE

- Equal amounts butter and oil, as needed
- 3 whole chicken breasts, boned, skinned, split and pounded thin
- Salt and pepper, as desired
- 10–12 water chestnuts
  For Liberal Diet, substitute 2 slices gluten bread.
- ¼ tsp. onion powder
- 1½ cups chicken broth
- ⅓ cup dry white wine
- 1½ tsp. dry mustard
- 2 dashes Tabasco sauce
- 1 tsp. lemon juice
- 1 tsp. Worcestershire sauce
- 3 Tbsp. butter
- ½ cup heavy cream

Heat butter and oil in frying pan. Season chicken with salt and pepper. Fry until tender and golden brown. Combine water chestnuts, onion powder, half of broth, wine, mustard, Tabasco, lemon juice, Worcestershire sauce and butter in blender until smooth. Pour into saucepan and add cream and remaining broth. Stir as sauce simmers 8 min. Do not allow to boil. Spoon over chicken.

Serves 4–6.

TERIYAKI CHICKEN

1 broiler-fryer, cut up
Pepper, as desired
Oregano, as desired
Garlic powder, as desired
½ cup Teriyaki sauce
⅓ cup oil
1 tsp. lemon juice
Sugar substitute equivalent to 1 tsp. sugar

Season chicken with pepper, oregano and garlic powder. Combine remaining ingredients. Place chicken pieces in shallow baking pan and pour Teriyaki mixture over top. Bake at 350 degrees for 30 min. Turn and bake for an additional 25–30 min., or until done as desired.

Serves 4.

CHICKEN PARMESAN

1 cup sunflower kernels
For Liberal Diet, substitute 1 cup Oven-Dried Gluten Bread Crumbs, p. 143.
½ cup Parmesan cheese, grated
4 whole chicken breasts, boned, skinned, pounded thin and split
1 egg, slightly beaten
Equal amounts butter and oil, as needed
2 cups Italian Spaghetti Sauce (p. 57)
8 oz. mozzarella cheese, sliced
½ cup Parmesan cheese, grated

Crush sunflower kernels in blender until they are the texture of fine bread crumbs. Combine with ½ cup Parmesan cheese. Dip chicken pieces in egg, then bread with nut mixture. Set aside on wax paper for 10 min. Fry chicken in butter and oil until golden brown. Spoon layer of sauce into baking dish. Layer 4 pieces of chicken over sauce. Place a slice of mozzarella cheese over each piece. Repeat layer of chicken and top each with a slice of cheese. Pour on remaining sauce and sprinkle with ½ cup Parmesan cheese. Bake at 350 degrees for 15–20 min. or until cheese melts and sauce bubbles.

Variation: Use veal in place of chicken.

Serves 6.

CHICKEN CACCIATORE

- 4–6 whole chicken breasts, boned, pounded and split
- Oil
- ½ cup tomato paste
- 1 (1 lb., 12 oz.) can whole tomatoes
- ⅓ cup liquid from canned tomatoes
- ⅓ cup green pepper, diced
- ½ tsp. parsley flakes
- ¾ tsp. garlic powder
- ¼ tsp. oregano
- ½ tsp. basil
- ½ tsp. celery seeds
- ¼ tsp. salt
- ½ cup dry white wine
- ½ cup chives

Fry chicken breasts in oil until lightly browned on both sides. Drain and place in baking dish. Combine all remaining ingredients except wine and chives in blender container. Process until smooth. Add wine and chives. Pour sauce over chicken. Bake, covered, for 40 min. at 350 degrees or until chicken is tender.

Variation: Substitute veal for chicken.

Serves 6–8.

RED WINE CHICKEN LIVERS

1½ cups chives, chopped
¼ cup butter
1 lb. chicken livers, cut in half
½ tsp. salt
⅛ tsp. pepper
½ tsp. thyme
2½ Tbsp. dry red wine

Sauté chives in butter. Add livers and brown quickly. Add remaining ingredients and cook, covered, for 10 min.

Serves 4.

TURKEY À LA KING

2 hard-boiled eggs
⅓ cup pimiento, chopped
2 cups White Cream Sauce (p. 55)
6 lg. slices white meat turkey, cooked
Celery seeds

Add eggs and pimiento to White Cream Sauce. Heat in double boiler or stir constantly over low heat in saucepan. Spoon over hot turkey slices and sprinkle with celery seeds.

Suggestion: For Liberal Diet, place turkey over Gluten Egg Noodles before topping with sauce.

Serves 4–6.

TURKEY AMANDINE

1 (4 oz.) can sliced mushrooms
½ cup almonds, slivered
2 cups White Cream Sauce (p. 55)
6 lg. slices turkey, cooked

Mix mushrooms and almonds in White Cream Sauce. Heat slowly in saucepan, stirring constantly, or in double boiler. Spoon over hot turkey slices.

Suggestion: For Liberal Diet, arrange turkey over Gluten Egg Noodles and top with sauce.

Serves 4–6.

TURKEY ITALIA

2 Tbsp. Parmesan cheese, grated
2 Tbsp. Swiss cheese, grated
½ tsp. parsley, chopped
4 lg. slices turkey, cooked

Combine Parmesan cheese, Swiss cheese and parsley. Sprinkle over turkey slices and bake at 375 degrees until cheese bubbles.

Serves 2–4.

VEAL STROGANOFF

1½ lbs. veal, cut into bite-size pieces
1 tsp. salt
¼ tsp. pepper
5 Tbsp. butter
1 cup whole mushrooms
½ cup chives
½ cup chicken broth
1½ Tbsp. lemon juice
½ cup dry red wine
6 water chestnuts
For Liberal Diet, substitute 1 slice gluten bread.
½ cup sour cream
1–2 zucchini, sliced lengthwise and sautéed in butter
For Liberal Diet, substitute Gluten Egg Noodles, p. 142.

Season veal with salt and pepper. Brown in 3 Tbsp. butter and set aside. Sauté mushrooms and chives in remaining 2 Tbsp. butter. In blender container, combine chicken broth, lemon juice, wine and water chestnuts. Add to mushroom pan with sour cream. Add veal and simmer, but do not allow to boil. When hot, serve over sliced zucchini.

Serves 4.

VEAL PARMESAN

1 cup sunflower kernels
For Liberal Diet, substitute 1 cup Oven-Dried Gluten Bread Crumbs, p. 143.
½ cup Parmesan cheese, grated
8 veal cutlets, pounded thin
1 egg, slightly beaten
1 cup chives, chopped
1 tsp. garlic powder
⅛ tsp. onion powder
2 Tbsp. butter
2 cups Basic Tomato Sauce (p. 61)
1 (1 lb.) can whole tomatoes
1 tsp. thyme
1½ tsp. basil
½ tsp. salt
¼ tsp. pepper
Equal amounts butter and oil, as needed
8 oz. mozzarella cheese, sliced
½ cup Parmesan cheese, grated

Crush sunflower kernels in blender until they are the texture of fine bread crumbs. Combine with Parmesan cheese. Dip veal in egg, then bread with nut mixture. Set aside on wax paper. Sauté chives with garlic powder and onion powder in 2 Tbsp. butter. Add Tomato Sauce, tomatoes, thyme, basil, salt and pepper. Cover and simmer 10 min. Brown veal in butter and oil until both sides are golden brown. Cover bottom of baking dish with layer of sauce. Arrange half of veal in pan. Cover each cutlet with a slice of mozzarella cheese. Repeat veal and mozzarella cheese layers, spoon on remaining sauce and top with ½ cup Parmesan cheese. Bake at 350 degrees for 15 min., or until cheese melts and sauce is bubbling hot.

Variation: Use chicken breasts in place of veal.

Serves 6–8.

Desserts

So often the craving for sweets usually felt by hypoglycemics and often by dieters in general makes remaining faithful to a diet seem nearly impossible. Primarily for this reason it is vital to have this dessert section. Do not give up desserts!

The protein content of some of these cheese cakes and pies is high enough so that a helping can be counted as one of the six hypoglycemic meals. While cheese and cream pies can be made successfully without a crust (by turning the mixture into a buttered glass dish and baking as directed), some crust recipes for the strict dieters are included here.

Flavored diet gelatin may be sprinkled into cheese cakes. When this is done, slightly reduce amount of sugar substitutes.

Lemon extract is the best substitute for lemon juice in baked goods, but use it sparingly. It tends to taste bitter when the flavor is too strong. Increase the quantity of the sugar substitute or add vanilla extract if you like a very strong lemon flavor.

Use meringue shells (shaped with the back of a spoon) for seafood cups, tart shells and custard cups. Bake in slow oven until brown and stiff. Cool slowly.

CRUMB PIE CRUST

¾ cup sunflower kernels
For Liberal Diet, substitute Oven-Dried Gluten Bread Crumbs, p. 143.
1½ tsp. liquid sugar substitute equivalent to ¼ cup sugar
2 Tbsp. water

Crush sunflower kernels in blender until they are the texture of fine bread crumbs. Add sugar substitute and water. When mixed, press into 9-in. pie pan. Bake at 350 degrees for 10 min. Cool.

Makes 1 9-in. crust.

DELIGHTFULLY NUTTY PIE SHELL

½ cup sunflower kernels
For Liberal Diet, substitute Oven-Dried Gluten Bread Crumbs, p. 143.
½ cup walnuts, chopped fine
Sugar substitute equivalent to 1 cup sugar
1 tsp. baking powder
1 egg, beaten
1 tsp. vanilla extract

Crush sunflower kernels in blender until they are the texture of fine bread crumbs. In bowl, combine sunflower kernels, walnuts, sugar substitute and baking powder. Add vanilla to ¼ egg. Pour mixture into nut bowl and mix until all dry ingredients have been moistened. Press into greased 9-in. pie pan, building up sides. Bake at 400 degrees for 15 min. Cool.

Makes 1 9-in. shell.

PIE SHELL FOR ALL

¼ cup butter
Liquid sugar substitute equivalent to 1 tsp. sugar
¾ cup coconut, flaked

Melt butter and mix with sugar substitute and coconut. Press into a 9-in. pie pan and bake 20 min. at 325 degrees. Cool.

Makes 1 9-in. shell.

MITE CRYSTAL DESSERT TOPPING

Sprinkle diet gelatin of desired flavor directly from package over cakes, pies, custards and gelatin desserts. Add during last 5 min. of baking time or use as is on chilled or frozen desserts. It is sweet and colorful.

CREAM FROSTING

½ tsp. vanilla extract
Sugar substitute equivalent to 1 Tbsp. sugar
½ cup sour cream
¼ tsp. imitation flavoring, optional

Combine all ingredients and spread on cake or pie. Bake at 325 degrees for 6–7 min. until frosting sets and appears glazed. For thick layer over pie filling, double recipe.

Suggestions:

To create your own frostings, try adding flavored diet gelatin straight from the package to Cream Frosting.

Add ½–¾ tsp. rum, bourbon or cognac to Cream Frosting in place of imitation flavoring.

Fold in fruit bits and bake in custard cups.

Makes ½ cup.

STRAWBERRY CREAM TOPPING

⅓ cup fresh or frozen strawberries, sliced
¼ cup sour cream
Sugar substitute equivalent to 1 tsp. sugar

Mash all ingredients together with a fork, leaving small strings of strawberry intact in pink cream. Spoon over pancakes or waffles, or spread on French toast. This topping is also delicious spread on cheese cake.

Makes about ½ cup.

CINNAMON SPRINKLE

1 Tbsp. cinnamon
4 Tbsp. granulated sugar substitute

Mix and store in small, covered dish. Use with pancakes, in desserts and for baking.

VANILLA DESSERT SAUCE

¾ cup butter, soft
¾ cup heavy cream (Use light cream for thinner sauce.)
1½ tsp. vanilla extract
Sugar substitute, to taste

Combine all ingredients in blender and mix until smooth. Heat and serve over desired desserts.

Variations: Add imitation brandy, rum or almond.

Makes about 2½ cups.

LEMON RICH DREAM PIE

12 oz. cream cheese
2 eggs
Sugar substitute equivalent to ½–¾ cup sugar
1 tsp. lemon juice
1 tsp. lemon rind, grated
2 tsp. vanilla extract
1 Crumb Pie Crust, baked and cooled (p. 113)
4 drops yellow food coloring
1 cup Cream Frosting (p. 115)

Combine cream cheese, eggs, sugar substitute, lemon juice, lemon rind and vanilla. Pour into crust and bake at 300 degrees for 40 min. or until filling is no longer wet. Cool about 10 min. Add food coloring to Cream Frosting and spread over filling. Bake 7 min. at 325 degrees, or until frosting sets and has a glaze. Cool and refrigerate 5 hrs. before serving.

Makes 1 9-in. pie.

FRESH STRAWBERRY PIE

- 3 baskets fresh strawberries
- ½ envelope unflavored gelatin *or*
  ½ envelope strawberry-flavored diet gelatin
- 1 cup water
- Sugar substitute equivalent to ½ cup sugar
- 1 Crumb Pie Crust (p. 113) or Pie Shell for All (p. 114)
- Whipped cream

Mash ⅔ of 1 basket of strawberries. Dissolve gelatin over water and stir in sugar substitute and mashed strawberries. Fill pie shell with strawberries and pour gelatin mixture over top. Refrigerate. Top with whipped cream before serving.

Variations: For Liberal Diet, blueberries and boysenberries may be prepared in same manner to make fabulous pies. Pies may be made from drained, canned diet fruits. Apple is good also.

Makes 1 9-in. pie.

COCONUT COTTAGE CHEESE PIE

- 1 cup light cream
- 2 Tbsp. lemon juice
- 2 egg yolks
- 1 cup cottage cheese
- Sugar substitute equivalent to 3 Tbsp. sugar
- ½ tsp. coconut extract
- 1 Pie Shell for All, baked and cooled (p. 114)

Cream all ingredients well and turn into Pie Shell for All. Bake at 300 degrees for 20 min. Top with meringue, if desired. Toast lightly in oven; cool and chill.

Makes 1 9-in. pie.

DELECTABLE STRAWBERRY CHEESE CAKE

10 oz. cream cheese, softened
¾ cup sour cream
Sugar substitute equivalent to ½–¾ cup sugar
1 egg
1¼ tsp. vanilla extract
1½ cups strawberries, sliced
1 Crumb Pie Crust, baked and cooled (p. 113)
¼ tsp. strawberry extract
2 drops red food coloring
½ cup Cream Frosting (p. 115)

Mix cream cheese, sour cream, sugar substitute, egg and vanilla. Beat until smooth. Stir in strawberry slices and turn into Crust. Bake at 300 degrees for 35 min. Add strawberry extract and food coloring to Cream Frosting. Spread over cake when it has cooled for 10 min. Return to 325 degree oven for 6 min. or until frosting sets and has a glaze. Cool and chill 4 hrs. before serving.

Variation: This cake may be made without crust. Turn cheese mixture into a buttered baking pan and bake as above.

Makes 1 9-in. cake.

VANILLA CHEESE CAKE WITH FRUIT

Strawberries, mashed as desired for fruit layer
1 Crumb Pie Crust, baked and cooled (p. 113)
Sugar substitute equivalent to 1 cup sugar
4 (8 oz.) pkgs. cream cheese, softened
3 eggs
½ cup light cream
¼ tsp. vanilla extract

Spoon strawberries over crust. Mix sugar substitute thoroughly into cream cheese. Cream in eggs one at a time. Slowly mix in cream and vanilla. Carefully pour mixture over strawberries. Bake at 425 degrees for 30–35 min. with baking pan sitting in larger pan of water, as for custard.

Variations:

Replace vanilla with imitation flavoring of your choice.

Omit fruit layer and replace vanilla with imitation almond or coconut and top with nuts and shredded coconut.

For Liberal Diet, substitute 2 lg. mashed apples for strawberries and replace vanilla with 3 drops imitation rum. This APPLE-RUM CHEESE CAKE is delicious.

Makes 1 9-in. cake.

COCONUT MACAROONS

Sugar substitute, as desired
2 egg whites
12 walnuts, chopped
2 Tbsp. coconut, shredded

Beat sugar substitute in egg whites until stiff. Fold in nuts and coconut. Drop one tsp. at a time onto a non-stick cookie sheet. Brown lightly at 350 degrees.

Makes 1½ dozen cookies.

STRAWBERRY CHIFFON

1 envelope cherry diet gelatin
2 cups water
1 cup whipping cream
Sugar substitute equivalent to 1 tsp. sugar
16 strawberries

Prepare gelatin in water and chill until slightly thickened. Whip with cream, sugar substitute and strawberries. Spoon into individual dessert cups and chill.

Serves 4–6.

MINT CHIFFON

1 envelope lime diet gelatin
2 cups water
⅛ tsp. peppermint extract
1 cup whipping cream

Prepare gelatin in water. Chill until slightly thickened. Add peppermint extract to cream, then whip with gelatin. Spoon into dessert cups and chill.

Variations:

Use lemon diet gelatin and a few drops imitation lemon flavoring.

Substitute orange diet gelatin for lime and orange extract for peppermint.

Combine 2 fruit diet gelatins and flavor with imitation brandy or rum.

Spoon mixture into Crumb Pie Crust or Pie Shell for All. Top with heavy cream whipped with imitation flavoring.

Serves 4–6.

HEAVENLY RICOTTA CAKE

2 egg whites
2 tsp. vanilla extract
16 oz. ricotta cheese
2 egg yolks
¼ tsp. salt
Sugar substitute equivalent to 1 cup sugar
½ cup light cream
2 Tbsp. lemon juice
Strawberries, as needed
Sugar substitute, to taste

Beat egg whites with vanilla until frothy. Refrigerate. Combine cheese with yolks, salt, sugar substitute, cream and lemon juice. Fold in chilled egg whites. Turn into 10-in. buttered glass pan. Bake at 350 degrees for 1 hr., 10 min.

Spread strawberries mashed with sugar substitute in layer over cake and return to oven just long enough to warm topping. Serve hot or cold.

Suggestions:

Add ½ tsp. Cinnamon Sprinkle and a dash of allspice to cheese mixture and frost with Cream Frosting.

Use a pie crust from Dessert Section. Fill with the cheese mixture.

For Liberal Diet, substitute Cinnamon-Apple Topping for strawberries.

Serves 6.

BERRY CHEESE GEL

1 envelope strawberry or black cherry diet gelatin
2 cups water
3 oz. cream cheese, rolled into balls
½ cup walnuts, chopped fine
1 basket strawberries

Prepare gelatin with water and chill until syrupy. Roll cheese balls in walnuts and drop into gelatin. Add strawberries and chill.

Serves 4–6.

STRAWBERRY MERINGUE

2 egg whites
Sugar substitute, as desired
1 cup strawberries, crushed

Beat egg whites with sugar substitute until stiff. Fold in strawberries and chill in custard cups.

Variations:

Substitute any fruit pulp for strawberries.

Add imititation flavorings to egg whites, as desired.

Serves 4.

CUSTARD WITH STRAWBERRIES

4 eggs, slightly beaten
3 cups heavy cream
1 tsp. vanilla extract
Dash salt
Sugar substitute equivalent to ⅓ cup sugar
12 strawberries, sliced

Combine all ingredients except strawberries. Pour into 6 individual custard cups and place in larger pan of hot water. Bake at 350 degrees for 40 min. or until knife inserted in center comes out clean. Remove cups from water and cover generously with strawberries. Sprinkle with sugar substitute, if desired.

Variations: Reduce vanilla to ½ tsp. and add ¼–½ tsp. imitation strawberry flavoring.

Replace vanilla extract with pineapple flavoring.

Serves 6.

TANGY QUICK GELS

1 envelope unflavored gelatin
2 cups fruit diet soda

Soften gelatin with ½ cup soda. Bring to a boil, stirring constantly, until gelatin dissolves. Add remaining 1½ cups soda and chill.

Suggestions:

Use unflavored gelatin with required amount of fruit juices. Add sugar substitute as needed.

Use flavored diet gelatin with lemon-lime diet soda or diet ginger ale.

Add imitation fruit flavorings to unflavored gelatin and color with food coloring.

Gel cantaloupe balls and strawberries in choice of diet gelatin.

Serves 4.

PINK DREAM WHIP SHERBET

- ¼–⅓ cup heavy cream
- ¼ cup wild raspberry diet soda
- 5 ice cubes
- ¼ tsp. vanilla extract
- ¼ tsp. cherry extract
- Sugar substitute equivalent to 3 tsp. sugar
- 1 egg, optional

Blend all ingredients until frothy. May be served immediately or frozen in dessert cups until desired consistency is obtained.

Variations:

Substitute diet soda of choice for wild raspberry.
Use imitation flavorings of choice for wide variety.

Serves 2–4.

LEMON SNOW

- 1 envelope unflavored gelatin
- 1¼ cups lemon-lime diet soda
- Sugar substitute equivalent to ⅓ cup sugar
- 1 Tbsp. lemon rind, grated
- ¼ cup lemon juice *or*
- 2 Tbsp. lemon juice and 2 Tbsp. lime juice
- 2 egg whites

Soften gelatin over lemon-lime diet soda. Add sugar substitute and heat, stirring constantly, until gelatin dissolves. Blend in lemon rind and juice. Cool until mixture mounds when dropped from a spoon. Beat egg whites until soft peaks form. Gently blend gelatin mixture into egg whites until mixture holds its shape. Spoon into custard cups and chill until firm.

Serves 4–6.

SCANDINAVIAN STRAWBERRY RUM

1 envelope unflavored gelatin
¼ cup cold water
2 Tbsp. boiling water
5 egg yolks
¼ med. lemon
Sugar substitute equivalent to ¾ cup sugar
⅓ cup rum
5 egg whites
Whipped cream
Strawberries

In blender container, soften gelatin over cold water and add boiling water. Process at low speed until gelatin is dissolved. With blender running, add egg yolks and lemon. Gradually add sugar substitute and continue blending. When mixture is smooth, add rum and process 10 seconds. Beat egg whites until stiff and fold in blender mixture. Pour into chilled 2-qt. mold and chill. Serve with whipped cream and strawberries.

Serves 4–6.

HOT FRUIT MINI FROSTS

2½ cups strawberries
½ cup Cream Frosting

Divide strawberries into 4 custard cups. Cover with Cream Frosting and bake at 325 degrees until frosting is glazed and fruit is hot.

Variations: For Liberal Diet, substitute boysenberries, blueberries or blackberries for strawberries. Canned peaches, pears and apricots are delicious prepared this way. Use your imagination for flavoring Cream Frosting to complement fruit.

Serves 4.

VERY CREAMY ORANGE PUDDING

1 envelope orange diet gelatin
1 cup boiling water
1 cup cold water
¾ cup whipping cream
Sugar substitute equivalent to 4 tsp. sugar
1 tsp. vanilla extract

Dissolve gelatin in boiling water, add cold and stir. Chill until mixture begins to gel. Whip cream with remaining ingredients, add to gelatin and stir well. Chill until set in mold or individual dessert cups.

Serves 4.

PECAN CRUNCH CANDY

Sugar substitute (granulated) equivalent to 2 cups sugar
1 cup pecans, chopped
2–2½ Tbsp. cold water

Heat sugar substitute over medium heat, stirring constantly, until it begins to melt. Quickly add nuts, then water. Stir rapidly and turn out onto a well-buttered cookie sheet. Spread mixture to desired thickness. Cool and break into pieces.

Note: This mixture becomes hard immediately after water is added. Use greased spoon or spatula to spread. (If mixture remains too moist, too much water was added. Dry in broiler.)

Variations:

Any allowed chopped nuts may be used alone or in combination. Add a small amount of extra water when cooking nuts.

Cooled crunch can be crumbled and used as a dessert topping.

STRAWBERRY CHEESE ROYALE

1 envelope cherry diet gelatin
1 cup boiling water
½ cup cold water
1 cup cottage cheese
1 cup strawberries
Whole strawberries, for garnish

Dissolve gelatin in boiling water. Pour into blender container and add cold water, cottage cheese and 1 cup strawberries. Process until smooth. Pour into dessert cups and freeze. Garnish with whole strawberries and serve.

Serves 6.

DO-IT-YOURSELF POPSICLES

Banana:
½ cup water or lemon-lime diet soda
¾ tsp. banana flavoring
Sugar substitute equivalent to 1 tsp. sugar
1 drop yellow food coloring

Strawberry:
½ cup lemon-lime diet soda
¼ tsp. imitation strawberry flavoring
Sugar substitute, to taste
1 drop red food coloring

Pineapple:
½ cup lemon-lime diet soda
¼ tsp. imitation pineapple flavoring
1 drop yellow food coloring

Combine all ingredients for chosen flavor and pour mixture into freezing trays designed for popsicles. Freeze.

Suggestions:

When using sodas for freezing, leave approximately ¾ in. space for expansion. (I use diet sodas which I have left open until they become flat.)

Use imitation flavoring with any diet soda, sweeten to taste.

Freeze allowed juices and fruit purées. They are delicious!

Milk and cream may be mixed with vanilla extract, imitation maple or instant decaffeinated coffee. They freeze well and provide a change in flavor.

FROSTED WALNUTS

Sugar substitute equivalent to 1 cup sugar
¼ tsp. allspice
½ tsp. cinnamon
Dash salt
¼ cup water
1 cup walnuts, shelled and halved

Combine sugar substitute, allspice, cinnamon, salt and water in saucepan. Stir constantly while mixture heats to the boiling point. Over medium heat, cook without stirring until mixture appears stringy, about 1 min. Remove from heat and quickly stir in walnuts. Separate nuts, if desired, and remove to buttered cookie sheet. Cool.

Variations:

Any allowed nuts may be substituted for walnuts. Adjust seasoning to nuts being used.

Use ½ tsp. nutmeg in place of allspice.

DELICIOUS PEELED ALMONDS

Boiling water
1 lb. almonds, shelled
1½ Tbsp. butter
Salt, to taste

Pour boiling water over almonds and peel off skins. Melt butter in pan and add almonds. Stir constantly over low heat until browned. Remove to brown paper and cool. Salt to taste.

MIXED GARLIC NUTS

2 cups mixed nuts
½ tsp. garlic powder
2 Tbsp. butter

Combine nuts with garlic powder and butter. Heat, stirring constantly.

Drinks

Recipes for diet drinks of all types are readily available from many sources. I have shared only my favorites with you. The Coffee Snack Cooler is delicious, and I often substitute it for a solid snack at night. It goes well with cheese slices and is not too filling.

Drinks are fun to experiment with. Sugarless diet sodas, milk or cream and ice cubes may be combined very successfully in a blender. The result is a frothy shake. Be creative with your own combinations.

PINK DREAM WHIP

5 ice cubes
⅓ cup light cream
¼ cup wild raspberry diet soda
¼ tsp. imitation cherry flavoring
¼ tsp. vanilla extract
Sugar substitute equivalent to 3 tsp. sugar
1 egg

Blend first 6 ingredients until frothy. Add egg to mixture and process to combine thoroughly. Serve immediately.

Makes 1½ cups.

STRAWBERRY TREAT

4 ice cubes
½ cup black cherry diet soda
6–8 strawberries
Sugar substitute, to taste

Combine all ingredients in blender and process until foamy.

Suggestion: Try favorite allowed fruit with lemon-lime diet soda.

Makes 1½ cups.

COFFEE SNACK COOLER

5 ice cubes
½ cup, half light cream, half water
For Liberal Diet, substitute ½ cup milk.
1 tsp. vanilla extract
Sugar substitute equivalent to 4 tsp. sugar
1 tsp. instant decaffeinated coffee
1 egg

Combine all ingredients in blender and process until thick and frothy.

Makes 1½ cups.

CREAMY EGG NOG

3 egg yolks
Sugar substitute equivalent to 2 Tbsp. sugar
3 Tbsp. light rum
2 Tbsp. bourbon
Dash salt
1 cup, half light cream, half water
For Liberal Diet, substitute 1 cup milk.
½ cup heavy cream
3 egg whites
Nutmeg

Beat egg yolks and gradually add sugar substitute. Continue beating until yolks are thick. Add rum, bourbon, salt and light cream with water. Whip heavy cream and beat egg whites until stiff peaks form. Fold whipped cream and yolk mixture into egg whites. Serve in chilled glasses and sprinkle nutmeg on top.

Serves 4–6.

HIGH PROTEIN TOMATO COCKTAIL

1 cup tomato juice
½ cup cottage cheese
Dash onion powder
Dash salt
⅛ tsp. celery salt

Combine all ingredients in blender. Process until smooth and serve immediately.

Makes 1½ cups.

STRAWBERRY SHAKE

6–8 strawberries
¾ tsp. vanilla
2 cups, half light cream, half water
For Liberal Diet, substitute 2 cups milk.
1 egg
Sugar substitute, to taste

Combine all ingredients in blender and process until foamy.

Variation: Any allowed fruit may be used in place of strawberries.

Makes 3 cups.

Part Three

Recipes for the Liberal Diet

Hors d'Oeuvres and Baked Cheeses

PARMESAN CHEESE ROUNDS

1 cup mayonnaise
¼ cup onion, finely grated
2 Tbsp. Parmesan cheese, grated
8 slices gluten bread
Parmesan cheese, grated

Mix mayonnaise, onion and 2 Tbsp. cheese. Using cookie cutter, prepare 4 rounds per slice gluten bread. Spread very generously with mixture and sprinkle with Parmesan cheese. Broil until lightly browned.

Makes 32.

SPECTACULAR FONDUE ROSELLE

12 slices Stretch-Cut Gluten Bread (6 regular slices), p. 143.
1 lb. Tillamook or sharp cheddar cheese, grated
Dash salt
6 eggs, well beaten
2½ cups milk

Remove crust from all 12 slices of bread and cut each into 9 cubes. Cover bottom of casserole dish with layer of bread cubes. Layer ⅓ of cheese over cubes. Repeat layers 3 times. Add salt to eggs and mix with milk. Pour mixture over top layer in casserole. Toss in remaining bread cubes and press down to moisten. Refrigerate 3–5 hrs. Bake at 350 degrees for 1 hr. and serve immediately. This is a dish for company. It always receives raves!

Serves 6.

CHEDDAR CUSTARD

½ tsp. salt
2 eggs
¼ tsp. dry mustard
⅛ tsp. pepper
2 cups milk
2½ cups cheddar cheese, cut into cubes
4 slices gluten bread

Combine salt, eggs, mustard, pepper and milk in blender. Add cheese cubes and process until mixed thoroughly. Tear bread into small pieces and mix well with cheese mixture. Pour into greased casserole dish placed in larger pan of hot water and bake at 350 degrees for 1 hr. or until knife inserted in center comes out clean.

Serves 6.

CHEESE SOUFFLÉ WITH BUTTERMILK

¼ cup butter
¼ cup gluten flour
1 cup buttermilk
1 cup sharp cheddar cheese, grated
¾ tsp. salt
Dash cayenne
¼ tsp. onion powder
6 eggs, separated and beaten

Melt butter. Stir in flour and slowly add buttermilk. Stir in cheese, salt, cayenne and onion powder. Add egg yolks and allow to cool. Fold in egg whites and turn into buttered casserole dish. Bake 45 min. at 350 degrees.

Serves 4–5.

PIGS IN A PASTRY BLANKET

Gluten Pasta (p. 142)
1 egg white
12 cocktail franks

Thoroughly brush baked Pasta on both sides with egg white. Cut into 12 elongated triangles. Place 1 frank on each triangle at base and roll up. Press seams to secure, using additional egg white if necessary. Place them on buttered cookie sheet and bake at 450 degrees for 8–10 min.

Makes 12.

Soups, Salads and Dressings

CLAM CHOWDER

2 cups White Cream Sauce (p. 55)
1 (10 oz.) can clams, minced, with liquid
⅓ cup onions, diced
½ cup celery, diced
½ cup carrots, diced
Dash Worcestershire sauce
Dash pepper
¼ tsp. thyme

Combine all ingredients in double boiler and heat slowly until vegetables are tender.

Variations: Substitute oysters for clams or combine both.

Serves 4.

FRENCH ONION SOUP

3 cups yellow onion, sliced thin
2 Tbsp. butter
1 Tbsp. oil
1 qt. beef bouillon, hot
1 tsp. salt
½ tsp. pepper
1½ Tbsp. gluten flour
½ cup dry white wine
¼ tsp. sage
1 bay leaf

Sauté onion in butter and oil until tender. Add to bouillon with salt, pepper, flour, wine and sage. Place bay leaf on top and simmer, covered, for 20 min.

Serves 6.

ONION SOUP FONDUE

½ cup Parmesan cheese, grated
2 qts. French Onion Soup (p. 138)
6–8 slices Garlic Bread (p. 145)
6–8 slices Monterey Jack cheese or other mild cheese

Add Parmesan cheese to soup and heat to boiling. Place 1 slice Garlic Bread in each serving bowl. Lay 1 slice cheese over each slice of bread. Fill each bowl with boiling soup. Serve immediately.

Serves 6–8.

CREAM OF CARROT SOUP

1 cup chicken stock
2 cups carrots, diced
2 whole cloves
Pinch salt
2 cups White Cream Sauce, medium (p. 55)

Combine chicken stock, carrots, cloves and salt in blender and mix until smooth. Stir into White Cream Sauce and heat slowly. Do not allow to boil.

Serves 3–4.

CREAMED PEA SOUP

1 cup peas
2 cups White Cream Sauce (p. 55)
⅓ cup onion, diced
½ tsp. salt
¼–½ tsp. white pepper
¼ cup celery, diced

Combine all ingredients in blender and mix until smooth. Heat gently but do not allow to boil.

Serves 2–3.

ZINGY CHICKEN SALAD

1 cup sour cream
¼ tsp. salt
½ cup celery, chopped
½ cup canned mushrooms, sliced
6–8 grapefruit sections, diced
¼ cup almonds, chopped or slivered
2 cups chicken, cooked and diced
Lettuce beds
⅓ cup stuffed olives

Combine sour cream, salt, celery, mushrooms, grapefruit, almonds and chicken. Place on lettuce beds and top with olives.

Serves 4.

CARAWAY COTTAGE SLAW

¾ cup cottage cheese
¾ cup sour cream
1 tsp. onion juice
½ tsp. salt
1 Tbsp. lemon juice
½ tsp. pepper
1 tsp. caraway seeds
½ tsp. celery seeds
3 cups red cabbage, shredded fine
1 cup apples, peeled, cored and diced
⅓ cup green pepper, chopped

Combine cottage cheese and sour cream. Add onion juice, salt, lemon juice, pepper, caraway and celery seeds. Mix well. Combine cabbage, apples and green pepper. Mix with cottage dressing and chill.

Serves 5–6.

GREEN GODDESS DRESSING FOR SALAD

1 cup mayonnaise
½ tsp. anchovy paste
½ cup parsley, chopped
⅓ cup onion, diced
⅛ tsp. garlic powder
2 Tbsp. tarragon vinegar
¼ cup cider vinegar
1 Tbsp. lemon juice
½ cup heavy cream

Combine all but last 2 ingredients in blender and mix until smooth. Add lemon juice and cream. Blend thoroughly.

Makes 1 pint.

ROQUEFORT DRESSING

2 oz. Roquefort cheese
2 Tbsp. boiling water
1 small clove garlic, minced
½ tsp. onion, grated
Dash Tabasco sauce
½ tsp. Worcestershire sauce
½ cup buttermilk
1 cup mayonnaise

Dissolve cheese in water and allow to stand ½ hr. Stir in remaining ingredients and refrigerate, covered, for at least 12 hrs.

Makes 1 pint.

Pastas

If you are on the Liberal Diet and therefore able to make use of this section, you should realize that these are the things which make *your* diet seem unlike most diets. Being able to eat noodles, croutons and pancakes should be well worth the time and effort spent on their preparation.

GLUTEN PASTA

- 2 slices gluten bread
- 2 eggs
- ⅛ tsp. salt
- ¼ cup milk
- ¼ cup light cream

Blend all ingredients in blender. Grease cookie sheet generously with butter or margarine. (It is best to use non-stick. However, if it is not available to you, the following instructions will enable you to prepare Gluten Pasta on any cookie sheet.) Place empty greased cookie sheet in 425 degree oven for 3½ min. Remove when butter bubbles and has just barely turned brown. Pour all batter except 2 Tbsp. onto sheet while rotating it so that batter sets evenly. Bake 10 min. or until pasta is glossy and has formed large air bubbles. Lightly browned edges should have pulled away slightly from sides of sheet. Flip upside down over bread board. Cool.

GLUTEN LINGUINE

Follow recipe for Gluten Pasta (above). Using pizza slicer or very sharp knife, cut ¼-in. strips all the way across width of pasta. Separate and use as desired.

GLUTEN EGG NOODLES

Prepare Gluten Pasta recipe. Use pizza cutter or sharp knife to cut ½-in. or ¾-in. noodles across width of baked pasta. Separate.

MOCK GLUTEN RICE

Follow recipe for Gluten Pasta. When done, slice length of pasta as thinly as possible with a pizza knife, cutter or very sharp kitchen knife. Then slice width as thinly as possible. Gather up tiny pieces and use in recipes calling for rice.

STRETCH-CUT GLUTEN BREAD

Using a very sharp knife, slice one flat piece of gluten bread horizontally through the center to divide it into two very thin slices.

Thin slices may be used for sandwiches. When toast is desired, slice after toasting. Very thin slices tend to burn easily.

GLUTEN BREAD CRUMBS

Place toasted, cooled bread in blender and crumble. Store in jar with tight-fitting lid in refrigerator.

OVEN-DRIED GLUTEN BREAD CRUMBS

Bake cut-up slices of gluten bread at 350 degrees for 8 min., then at 500 degrees until hard and dark golden brown. Do not allow to burn as flavor is affected. Crush in blender or with a rolling pin. Place in a jar with a tight lid and refrigerate.

BUTTERED GLUTEN CRUMBS

Bake as for Oven-Dried Gluten Bread Crumbs. Crush and put crumbs into a bowl. Drip melted butter over them and toss with a fork. Pour off excess butter, if any. Store in jar in refrigerator.

CROUTONS PARMESAN

1 slice gluten bread
2 Tbsp. butter
Dash onion powder
¼ tsp. garlic powder
1¼ tsp. Parmesan cheese, grated

Slice bread 5 times each way. Melt butter in pot and add remaining ingredients. Mix thoroughly. Toss bread squares into pot. Mix quickly until all sides have been saturated and entire mixture has been absorbed. Remove squares to baking pan. Place in 350 degree oven for 8 min. to dry; then broil lightly on all sides. Cool croutons and store in refrigerator in covered jar.

Makes 36 croutons.

ITALIAN CROUTONS

1 slice gluten bread
2 Tbsp. butter
¼ tsp. garlic powder
1¼ tsp. Romano cheese, grated
⅛ tsp. salt

Prepare croutons following directions for Croutons Parmesan.

BLEU CHEESE CROUTONS

1 slice gluten bread
2½ Tbsp. butter
1½ tsp. bleu cheese, crumbled
Dash salt

Prepare croutons following directions for Croutons Parmesan.

FRENCH CROUTONS

1 slice gluten bread
2¼ Tbsp. coconut oil

Prepare croutons following directions for Croutons Parmesan.

GARLIC BREAD

8 slices gluten bread
½ cup butter
1 tsp. garlic powder
1½ Tbsp. Parmesan cheese, grated
¼ tsp. onion powder
Paprika, if desired to color

Toast bread lightly. Melt butter in small, shallow pan. Stir in garlic powder, cheese and onion powder. Using fork, dip each slice of toast in butter mixture until it is saturated. Place on broiling pan and sprinkle lightly with paprika. Broil until bubbly brown. Serve.

Variations:

Replace Parmesan cheese with grated Romano.

Mix half Parmesan and half Romano for an interesting change in flavor.

CINNAMON-APPLE PANCAKES

1 slice gluten bread
1 egg
2 Tbsp. milk
2 Tbsp. light cream
¼ recipe Cinnamon-Apple Topping (p. 180)

Combine first 4 ingredients in blender and mix until smooth. Add Cinnamon-Apple Topping and process until slightly lumpy. Cook as directed for Breakfast Pancakes (p. 150) and top with applesauce, canned without sugar, or with Cinnamon Sprinkle.

Makes 4–6 pancakes.

FRENCH PANCAKES

¼ cup + 1 Tbsp. milk
2 eggs
1 slice gluten bread
¼ tsp. salt
½ tsp. melted butter
Sugar substitute equivalent to 1 tsp. sugar
Cinnamon-Apple Topping (p. 180)

Combine first 6 ingredients in blender and mix until creamy. Heat butter in pan. Pour thin pancake into center of pan. Remove from heat while rotating pan to cover bottom evenly. Return to heat for 20 seconds or until pancake stiffens slightly. Flip and fry 15–20 seconds. Turn out onto wax paper, spread with Cinnamon-Apple Topping and roll up. Pancakes may be topped with melted butter and sugar substitute. These are very delicate, so handle carefully.

Suggestions:

Berry toppings are delicious on these.
Use as crepes for spectacular seafood roll-ups.
Roll with cooked vegetables and top with a cream soup.

Makes 4–6 pancakes.

SPICE PANCAKES

1 slice gluten bread
1 egg
⅛ cup milk
⅛ cup light cream
⅛ tsp. allspice
Pinch clove and nutmeg
Sugar substitute equivalent to 1 tsp. sugar

Blend all ingredients and process in blender until batter is creamy. Pour into hot buttered pan and cook as directed for Breakfast Pancakes (p. 150). Top with butter and Cinnamon Sprinkle.

Makes 4–6 pancakes.

BUTTERMILK PANCAKES

1 egg
¼ cup buttermilk
1 tsp. butter
1 slice gluten bread
⅛ tsp. salt
Sugar substitute equivalent to 1 tsp. sugar

Put all ingredients in blender and mix until smooth. Pour or spoon pancakes into frying pan bubbling with melted butter. Turn only once, when pancakes are golden brown. Top with Maple Syrup, Fruit Topping, Cinnamon Sprinkle or sugarless jam.

Makes 4–6 pancakes.

ORANGE HIGH-RISE PANCAKES

4 tsp. unsweetened orange juice
¼ tsp. cinnamon
¼ tsp. salt
⅛ tsp. baking soda
½ tsp. butter, soft
1 slice gluten bread
1 egg yolk
1 Tbsp. milk
2 Tbsp. light cream
1 egg white
Sugar substitute equivalent to 3 tsp. sugar
Orange Sauce (p. 181)

Put first 9 ingredients in the blender and process at low speed stopping often to lower moist crumbs into the blades. Continue mixing until batter is smooth. Beat egg white and sugar substitute until it is stiff. Fold white into batter. Cook over medium heat in buttered frying pan until done. Top with Orange Sauce.

Makes 4–6 pancakes.

STRAWBERRY PANCAKES

1 slice gluten bread
1 egg
¼ cup buttermilk
Sugar substitute equivalent to 1 tsp. sugar
3 fresh strawberries *or*
3 strawberries frozen without sugar, thawed
Strawberry Cream Topping (p. 115)

Put first 4 ingredients in a blender and process until smooth. Add strawberries and blend on medium speed until strawberries are in small bits. Cook as directed for Buttermilk Pancakes (p. 147) and top with Strawberry Cream.

Variations: Blueberries, blackberries or raspberries may be substituted for strawberries or ¾ of an apricot, canned without sugar, may be used. They are all delicious topped with fruit jam or Strawberry Syrup.

Makes 4–6 pancakes.

RICOTTA PUFFS

1 egg white
1 slice gluten bread
1 egg yolk
⅛ cup light cream
⅛ cup milk
Dash salt
¼ tsp. baking powder
Sugar substitute equivalent to 2 tsp. sugar
3 Tbsp. ricotta cheese

Beat egg white until soft peaks form. Refrigerate. Combine all remaining ingredients, except cheese, in blender. Process until smooth. Add cheese and mix well. Pour into bowl and fold in chilled egg white. Drop onto hot buttered frying pan. Brown lightly, turning only once. Cakes may be made by dropping batter onto greased cookie sheet and baking at 350 degrees until bottom browns lightly.

Suggestions:

Top with Vanilla or Strawberry Topping. Use for dessert.
Spread with Strawberry Jam.
Add orange juice to batter before baking.
Add imitation flavoring to batter.

Makes 10.

FLUFFY FRENCH TOAST

1 egg
1 Tbsp. light cream
Dash salt and pepper
Butter
2 slices gluten bread
Cream cheese
Cinnamon Sprinkle (p. 115)

Beat egg with cream, salt and pepper until frothy. Melt generous amount of butter in frying pan and heat until it bubbles vigorously. Dip bread slices in mixture and coat with butter by dropping on hot pan. Turn immediately, before browning occurs. Add additional butter, cover and cook until golden brown. Turn slices and replace cover to complete cooking. Cook slightly and spread generously with cream cheese. Top with Cinnamon Sprinkle.

Variations:

Add vanilla or any desired extract to egg mixture before dipping bread.
Add cinnamon or Cinnamon Sprinkle to egg mixture.

Serves 1–2.

BREAKFAST PANCAKES

2 Tbsp. apple, peeled and diced, optional
1 slice gluten bread
1 egg
2 Tbsp. milk
Sugar substitute equivalent to 1 tsp. sugar
2 Tbsp. light cream
⅛ tsp. Cinnamon Sprinkle (p. 115)

Put all ingredients in a blender and process until batter is smooth. Pour pancakes into a hot buttered pan or onto a griddle and turn when bubbles appear. Cook only once on each side. Brown on second side and serve. Top with Apricot Preserves, Cinnamon-Apple Topping or Maple Syrup.

Variations:

Include 1½ tsp. diced ham or bacon bits in batter.
Mix 1 Tbsp. finely chopped onion into batter.

Makes 4–6 pancakes.

SOUR CREAM PANCAKES

1 slice gluten bread
⅛ cup milk
⅛ cup light cream
1 egg
2 tsp. cottage cheese
2 Tbsp. sour cream
Sugar substitute equivalent to 1½ tsp. sugar

Blend all ingredients at high speed until mixed thoroughly. Let stand 5 min., then reblend for only a second or two. Pour into a moderately hot buttered pan. Cook as directed for Breakfast Pancakes (p. 150) but watch these carefully as they get done quickly. Top with Cinnamon Sprinkle.

Makes 4–6 pancakes.

VANILLA FLUFF PANCAKES

1 egg, separated
Sugar substitute equivalent to 2½ tsp. sugar
2 Tbsp. milk
2 Tbsp. light cream
1 slice gluten bread
1 tsp. vanilla flavoring

Combine egg yolk, sugar substitute, milk, cream and bread in blender and mix until smooth. Beat egg white and vanilla until peaks form. Fold batter into egg white. Cook over moderate heat until golden brown. Top with favorite fruit topping or Maple-Butter Syrup.

Makes 4–6 pancakes.

Vegetables

FRUIT-VEGETABLE STUFFING

2 apples, peeled and sliced thin
1 med. onion, sliced thin
1 head cabbage, shredded
2 oranges, with peel, sliced thin
1¾ cups celery, chopped
¼ cup butter or margarine
1 tsp. ground ginger
1½ Tbsp. soy sauce
½ cup Oven-Dried Gluten Bread Crumbs (p. 143)

Cook apples, onion, cabbage, oranges and celery in butter for 5–6 min. Add ginger, soy sauce and Crumbs. Stir well, cover and remove from heat. Allow to steam 4–5 min. Use to stuff Cornish game hens or turkey.

Makes 6–8 cups.

BEET VEGETABLE TOPPING

1 cup beets, minced
1 cup sour cream

Heat beets. Add sour cream and heat slowly, stirring constantly. Do not allow to boil. Serve over green vegetables.

Makes 2 cups.

SOUR CREAM BEETS

2 tsp. vinegar
½ tsp. salt
Dash cayenne
2 tsp. leeks, minced
¼ cup sour cream
Sugar substitute equivalent to 1 tsp. sugar
2½ cups beets, cooked and halved

Combine vinegar, salt, cayenne, leeks, sour cream and sugar substitute. Add cooked beets and stir. Simmer until hot.

Suggestion: Do not discard beet tops! They are extremely nutritious. Tear them into pieces and include in beet recipes.

Serves 4.

CABBAGE 'N CLOVES

¼ cup water
1 med. red cabbage, shredded
1 apple, cored and chopped
1 tsp. salt
1/3 cup vinegar
Sugar substitute equivalent to ¼ cup sugar
7 cloves

Mix all ingredients in a saucepan. Simmer, covered, for 20 min. Remove cloves and serve.

Serves 4–6.

MOZZARELLA ARTICHOKE HEARTS

1 (6 oz.) can artichoke hearts
1 (10 oz.) pkg. frozen chopped spinach, heated through
1 Tbsp. parsley, chopped
1 cup sour cream
½ cup mozzarella cheese, grated

Drain artichoke hearts. Cover with spinach in baking dish. Mix parsley into sour cream and spread over spinach. Sprinkle cheese over top and bake at 350 degrees for 25 min.

Serves 6.

REGAL KING CRAB ARTICHOKES

6 lg. artichokes, with stems and tops removed
½ cup boiling water
2 (7¾ oz.) cans king crab meat, membranes removed
1 tsp. salt
2 tsp. white horseradish
Salsa Jalapeña (hot red chili relish), to taste
1½ cups sour cream
Parsley, chopped

Put artichokes, petals down, into water; cover and steam 25–30 min. Drain, cool and remove centers. Flake crab meat and mix with salt, horseradish, Salsa Jalapeña and sour cream. Spread mixture on leaves and fill center cup. Garnish with parsley.

Serves 6.

CARROTS IN WINE

2 lbs. carrots, scraped and quartered
¼ cup butter
1 tsp. salt
⅛ tsp. pepper
Sugar substitute equivalent to ¼ tsp. sugar
½ cup dry red wine
Parsley, minced

Sauté carrots in butter, turning until well coated. Sprinkle with salt, pepper and sugar substitute. Add wine and simmer for 5 min. Add water to cover carrots and simmer, covered, for an additional 15–25 min. Remove cover and cook over medium heat until most of liquid has evaporated. Sprinkle with parsley and serve.

Serves 8.

CARROT BAKE PUFF

3 cups carrots, scraped and cut
1 small onion, diced
½ cup chicken stock
2 eggs
3 Tbsp. butter, softened
½ tsp. salt
2 slices gluten bread, torn in pieces

Place all ingredients in blender and chop. Pour into baking dish and bake 1 hr. at 350 degrees.

Serves 4.

MAPLED CARROTS

½ lb. carrots, cooked
2 Tbsp. butter
¼ cup Maple Syrup (p. 62)
Brown sugar substitute equivalent to 2 tsp. sugar

Layer carrots in buttered baking dish. Mix butter, Syrup and brown sugar substitute in bowl. Spoon over carrots. Broil, turning frequently to glaze.

Serves 2.

BATTER-FRIED MUSHROOMS

2 doz. mushrooms caps
Gluten Pasta, uncooked batter (p. 142)
1 cup Oven-Dried Gluten Bread Crumbs (p. 143)
Oil for deep frying

Wash mushrooms quickly and dry on paper towels. Dip each first into Gluten Pasta batter then into Crumbs. Drop into very hot, deep fat. Turn each when brown. Fry on second side. Drain and serve hot.

Serves 4–6.

DEEP-FRIED ONION RINGS

3 lg. onions
1–2 eggs
Sugar substitute equivalent to 1 tsp. sugar
⅔ cup Oven-Dried Gluten Bread Crumbs (p. 143)
½ tsp. salt
¼ tsp. pepper
Oil

Peel onions and slice into ¼–½-in.-thick slices. Discard top and bottom slices. Separate remaining slices into rings. Beat eggs, add sugar substitute. Combine Crumbs with salt and pepper. Dip rings first into egg mixture, then coat well with Crumb mixture. Drop into hot, deep oil and fry until golden brown. Drain.

Serves 4–6.

ZESTY STUFFED ONIONS

3 Spanish onions, peeled and cut in half
1½ cups Gluten Bread Crumbs (p. 143)
1¼ cloves garlic, minced
2 Tbsp. parsley, chopped
⅛ tsp. oregano
¼ tsp. salt
2 Tbsp. butter, melted
2 Tbsp. Parmesan cheese, grated
1½ Tbsp. melted butter
1½ Tbsp. Parmesan cheese, grated

Remove center part of onions, creating shells. Chop 2 Tbsp. of removed centers and add Crumbs, garlic, parsley, oregano, salt, 2 Tbsp. butter and 2 Tbsp. cheese. Toss until mixed. Fill onions with mixture and top with 1½ Tbsp. butter and 1½ Tbsp. cheese. Bake, covered, at 375 degrees for 25 min. or until onions are tender.

Serves 6.

BATTER-FRIED ONION RINGS WITH SWISS CHEESE SAUCE

3 lg. onions
1 cup Gluten Pasta batter (p. 142)
1 cup Swiss Cheese Sauce (p. 59)
Oil

Prepare onions as for Deep-Fried Onion Rings (p. 156). Dip rings into Pasta batter and drop into very hot oil. Brown well on both sides. Drain and pour Cheese Sauce over rings. Serve immediately.

Serves 6–8.

SPICE-CARROT SOUFFLÉ

¾ lb. carrots, cooked and diced
⅔ cup White Cream Sauce, medium (p. 55)
Brown sugar substitute equivalent to 2 tsp. sugar
Sugar substitute equivalent to 1 tsp. sugar
2 eggs, separated
Salt and pepper, as desired
Pinch allspice
Pinch nutmeg

Mix ½ lb. carrots with White Cream Sauce in blender until smooth. Stir in remaining ¼ lb. carrots, sugar substitutes, beaten egg yolks, salt, pepper, allspice and nutmeg. Beat egg whites until stiff but still moist. Fold into carrot mixture. Pour into buttered baking dish and bake at 375 degrees for 25–30 min. or until knife inserted in center comes out clean.

Note: This soufflé can be made successfully in individual custard cups.

Serves 4–6.

PARMESAN ONIONS IN WINE SAUCE

5–6 med. onions, sliced and separated into rings
½ tsp. salt
½ tsp. pepper
Sugar substitute equivalent to ½ tsp. sugar
½ cup butter
½ cup dry red wine
Parmesan cheese, grated

Season onion rings with salt, pepper and sugar substitute. Sauté in butter until barely tender. Add wine and simmer 2 min. Remove onions and sauce to serving dish and sprinkle Parmesan cheese on top.

Serves 6–8.

BROCCOLI ROULADES MARINARA

1 (10 oz.) pkg. frozen chopped broccoli
¾ cup ham, diced
Gluten Pasta, baked (p. 142)
1 egg white
2½–3 cups Marinara Sauce (p. 56)

Cook broccoli and drain. Mix with ham. Brush Pasta generously on both sides with egg white and cut into 6 rectangles. Spoon small amount of broccoli mixture onto each rectangle and spread to within ½ in. of edges. Roll up and press to seal, using additional egg white if necessary. Place rolls in shallow buttered baking dish and bake at 450 degrees until stuffing is hot and rolls are golden brown. Spoon Marinara Sauce over rolls.

Suggestions:

Many vegetables lend themselves well to this recipe. Try using squash or spinach in place of broccoli.

Almost any leftover meat may be cut up and used to add new flavor to familiar vegetables.

Top roulades with Cheese Sauce, Swiss Cheese Sauce or Tomato-Cheese Sauce.

Serves 6.

STUFFED APPLES

7–8 oz. yellow squash, diced
½ tsp. nutmeg
¾ tsp. cinnamon
6 lg. red apples
⅓ cup lemon juice
Brown sugar substitute equivalent to ⅓ cup sugar
½ can lemon-lime diet soda

Cook squash until hot. Mix with nutmeg and cinnamon. Peel and core apples. Dip into lemon juice and sprinkle heavily with sugar substitute. Stuff cored apples with squash mixture. Place in baking dish in 350 degree oven for 1 hr. Mix 1 Tbsp. lemon juice with diet soda and use to baste apples during cooking.

Serves 6.

ORIGINAL FRIED TOMATO SLICES

4 medium tomatoes, firm
½ cup powdered non-fat milk
1½ tsp. salt
2 eggs
Sugar substitute equivalent to 1 tsp. sugar
1 cup Oven-Dried Gluten Bread Crumbs (p. 143)

Wash, dry and cut tomatoes into ½-in.-thick slices. Discard top and bottom slices. Combine dry milk and salt. Beat eggs with sugar substitute. Dip tomato slices into powdered milk, coating thoroughly; then dip into egg mixture and finally into Crumbs. Drop slices into hot oil and cook until golden brown on both sides.

Serves 6.

Entrees

ITALIAN SPAGHETTI WITH MEAT SAUCE

1 lb. ground beef
Salt, pepper and garlic powder, as desired
4½ cups Italian Spaghetti Sauce (p. 57)
Double recipe Gluten Linguine (p. 142)
Parmesan cheese, grated

Season ground beef with salt, pepper and garlic powder. Crumble beef while pan-browning. Add to Italian Spaghetti Sauce and cook over low heat for 25 min. Meanwhile, prepare Gluten Linguine. When sauce is done, spoon over noodles and serve with grated Parmesan cheese sprinkled on top.

Serves 3–4.

RAVIOLI WITH MEAT SAUCE

Gluten Pasta, baked (p. 142)
4½ cups Italian Spaghetti Sauce (p. 57)
1 lb. ground beef
Salt, pepper and garlic powder, as desired
1 egg white

Cut width of baked Pasta in half. Place one half Pasta over other half. Cut with pizza cutter or very sharp kitchen knife into 2-in. squares by slicing first one way then the other. Brown seasoned meat in frying pan. With a spoon, place approximately 2 Tbsp. meat on lower piece of ravioli square. Place top piece over it and seal by placing small amount of egg white around all four edges of ravioli and between layers at edges, then pinch. Put sealed ravioli into a covered dish and bake at 350 degrees until hot. Meanwhile, heat Italian Spaghetti Sauce in a saucepan. When both ravioli and sauce are done, spoon sauce over ravioli and serve.

Serves 4.

FRENCH ONION MEAT LOAF WITH GRAVY

1 lb. ground beef
5 Tbsp. French Onion Soup (p. 138)
3 Tbsp. Gluten Bread Crumbs (p. 143)
Salt
Pepper
Garlic powder
1 medium onion, halved
1⅔ cups French Onion Soup (p. 138)
2 Tbsp. ketchup

Season meat with 5 Tbsp. French Onion Soup, Crumbs, salt, pepper and garlic powder. Form into a loaf and bake with onion at 400 degrees for 15 min. Drain. Add 1⅔ cups French Onion Soup and top loaf with ketchup. Lower oven to 350 degrees and continue baking for 40 min. or until done as desired.

Serves 4.

TACOS

1 lb. ground beef
1 small onion, chopped
1 tsp. salt
2 Tbsp. taco sauce *or*
Dash Tabasco sauce and 1 green chili, shredded
8–10 taco shells (or corn tortillas)
1 med. tomato, diced
¾ cup lettuce, shredded
2 cups cheddar cheese, grated

Combine beef with onion, salt and taco sauce. Brown until crumbly. Bake taco shells according to package directions and stuff with meat mixture, tomato and lettuce. Top with generous layer of cheese.

Serves 4.

CHEESE AND TOMATO PIZZA

Pizza Sauce:

2 (1 lb.) cans Italian tomatoes, drained
1 Tbsp. liquid from canned tomatoes
2 Tbsp. tomato paste
1 Tbsp. bell pepper, diced
1 tsp. onions, chopped
1/16 tsp. oregano
⅛ tsp. garlic powder
Dash parsley flakes
4 oz. mozzarella cheese

Crust:

1 egg
Dash salt
¼ cup milk
1 slice gluten bread

Pre-heat oven at 425 degrees for 15 min. Generously grease 2 pie pans and place empty in pre-heated oven for 3 min. or until grease is very hot and ready to bubble, but not browned; or use non-stick pans for convenience. Blend crust ingredients in blender and process until smooth. Pour about 1 oz. into each hot pie pan and place in oven. Remove after 8–10 min. or when crust is stiff and looks glazed. Process all pizza sauce ingredients, except mozzarella cheese, in a blender. When mixed thoroughly, spoon 2 Tbsp. evenly over each pizza to within ½ in. of edges. Top each with 2 oz. mozzarella cheese, placed to within ½ in. of edges. Return pizzas to oven and bake until edges of crust are brown and cheese is completely melted.

Note: A large rectangular pizza can be made by doubling crust recipe and baking it on a cookie sheet.

Variations:

Prepare Cheese and Tomato Pizzas and top with sliced onion just before last baking.

Add bell pepper strips over mozzarella cheese.

Use mushrooms on top. Sprinkle with Parmesan cheese.

Cover with baby shrimp before last baking.
Cover cheese with bacon bits or any leftover meat bits.
Place anchovies on top.
Add clams over cheese.
Top with olives.
Prepare meatballs, slice and top pizzas.
Top with diced cold cuts.
Cover with lobster or flaked fish, and sprinkle grated Parmesan cheese on top.
Shrimp and crab make delicious additions.

Serves 2.

TAQUITOS WITH AVOCADO SAUCE

1 med. avocado, peeled
2 Tbsp. onion, diced
2 Tbsp. sour cream
5 Tbsp. water
¼ tsp. salt
Dash pepper
½ tsp. lemon juice
1/16 tsp. garlic powder
¾ tsp. Salsa Jalapeña (hot red chili relish)
6 corn tortillas
6 slices rare roast beef, sliced very thin
Oil

Combine avocado, onion, sour cream, water, salt, pepper, lemon juice, garlic powder and Salsa Jalapeña and mix in blender until smooth. Heat each tortilla on both sides over open flame. Place beef slice over tortilla and roll tightly. Secure with a toothpick. When all 6 have been completed, fry them in hot oil on all sides until browned and crisp. Remove and set at an angle so that oil drains out. Tilt in serving bowls with avocado sauce poured over ends.

Serves 3.

MEXICALE ENCHILADAS

4 corn tortillas
4 slices rare roast beef, sliced extra thin, *or* Browned ground beef
8 oz. sharp cheddar cheese, sliced
½ tsp. garlic powder
3 cups Basic Tomato Sauce (p. 61)
4 tsp. Salsa Jalapeña (hot red chili relish)
¼ cup onion, chopped
1 tsp. salt

Heat tortillas on both sides over open flame. Cover center third with meat. Layer cheese slices over meat (about 1 oz. per tortilla). Fold up sides and secure with toothpicks. Combine garlic powder, Tomato Sauce, Salsa Jalapeña, onion and salt. Pour small amount of sauce in bottom of baking pan. Place enchiladas in pan and cover each with about 2 Tbsp. sauce. Place remaining cheese on top and bake at 375 degrees until cheese inside melts.

Variations:
Gluten Pasta may be substituted for tortillas.
Add chopped olives to meat.

Makes 4.

HOT DOG CASSEROLE

12 all-beef frankfurters
2 cups Cheese Sauce (p. 58)
½ cup chives
Gluten Egg Noodles (p. 142)

Cut franks into bite-size pieces. Mix into Cheese Sauce and stir in chives. Mix with Noodles and put into buttered baking dish. Bake, covered, at 375 degrees until franks are thoroughly heated, about 20 min. Cover may be removed last 5 min. of baking to brown top, if desired.

Variation: Use Swiss Cheese Sauce for a change in flavor.

Serves 4.

PORK CHOPS WITH APPLE SAUERKRAUT

8 pork chops
Salt and pepper, as desired
Oil
1 large apple, diced
1 lb. cherry tomatoes
1 (1 lb., 12 oz.) can sauerkraut, drained
¼ tsp. sesame seeds
¼ tsp. caraway seeds
1 cup onion, diced

Season chops with salt and pepper. Brown on both sides in oil and drain, reserving 2 Tbsp. pan drippings. To drippings, add apple, tomatoes, sauerkraut, seeds and onion. Sauté until onion is tender. Spoon mixture into greased baking pan and arrange chops over top. Bake, covered, at 350 degrees for 35 min. or until chops are tender.

Serves 4.

SPICY APPLESAUCE SPARERIBS

3 lbs. spareribs
1½ Tbsp. salt
1¼ tsp. cinnamon
¼ tsp. cloves
¼ tsp. nutmeg
Sugar substitute equivalent to 3 Tbsp. sugar
1 cup applesauce, canned without sugar
¼ cup lemon juice

Season ribs with salt. Place in shallow, lined baking dish. Combine remaining ingredients and place over low heat. Brush ribs well with mixture and bake, brushing often, at 325 degrees for 1½ hrs.

Variation: This applesauce mixture is excellent brushed on pork chops, too.

Serves 6.

PORK WITH CHOW MEIN

2 pork loins
Teriyaki sauce
2 med. white onions, diced
¾–1 lb. mushrooms
1 Tbsp. oil
1 can bean sprouts
2 cans water chestnuts
1 pkg. pea pods
1 Tbsp. gluten flour

Marinate pork in Teriyaki sauce. Cook at 400 degrees for 30 min. Sauté onions and mushrooms in oil. Add bean sprouts and water chestnuts. Slice pork and cook pea pods. Add both to vegetable mixture and simmer. Stir in flour to thicken. Simmer 3 min. and serve.

Serves 8.

MILD MEATBALLS IN PEPPERCORN GRAVY

4 cups water
1 cup onion, minced
3 bay leaves
¼ cup lemon juice
½ tsp. allspice
7 peppercorns
1½ tsp. salt
1 lb. ground beef
¾ cup Gluten Bread Crumbs (p. 143)
¼ tsp. pepper
1 egg, slightly beaten
3 Tbsp. butter
Gluten flour
Gluten Egg Noodles (p. 142)

Boil water and add ⅓ cup onion, bay leaves, lemon juice, allspice, peppercorns and ¾ tsp. salt. Continue boiling about

10 min. Combine meat with remaining ⅔ cup onion, remaining ¾ tsp. salt, Crumbs, pepper and egg. Form into balls and drop into boiling liquid. Simmer 15–18 min. Remove meatballs and pour off liquid, reserving 2½ cups in saucepan. Pour off fat; if necessary, add butter and stir in gluten flour until gravy is of desired consistency. Add meatballs to gravy and serve over Gluten Egg Noodles.

Suggestion: Try gravy over meatloaf.

Serves 4.

FRUITY HAM BASTE

- 1 butt or shank cut ham
- 1 med. apple, peeled and cored
- Liquid from 2 cans diet apricots
- ⅛ tsp. imitation cherry flavoring
- Brown sugar substitute
- Cloves

Remove outer skin from ham and cut fat so that an even layer remains. Score. Combine apple, apricot liquid and cherry flavoring in blender and mix until smooth. Moisten ham with mixture and pat on brown sugar substitute. Arrange cloves on ham and place it in baking pan. Pour apple mixture in bottom of pan and bake at 350 degrees, basting often with mixture for 2 hrs., or until done as desired.

Variations: Any allowed canned diet fruit may be puréed, combined with can liquid and used for marinating and basting meats.

Serves 6–8.

FLOUNDER AMANDINE

2 eggs
1 Tbsp. milk
½ tsp. salt
1 Tbsp. lemon juice
1½ cups Gluten Bread Crumbs (p. 143)
3 Tbsp. dehydrated parsley flakes
2 lbs. flounder fillets
4 Tbsp. butter
½ cup almonds, slivered

Beat eggs with milk, salt and lemon juice. Combine Crumbs and parsley flakes. Dip fillets in egg mixture, then coat with Crumbs. Melt butter in pan and add fillets. Toss in almonds. Cook fillets 4 min. on each side, occasionally stirring almonds. Remove fish to serving plates and top with almonds.

Suggestion: This recipe lends itself well to many types of fish. Try your favorite for a new taste treat.

Serves 4.

WRAPPED SALMON LOAF SUPREME

Salmon loaf and Sauce as for Salmon Loaf Supreme (p. 93). Omit Crumbs from top.
Gluten Pasta (p. 142), baked only until set
1 egg
1 Tbsp. milk or light cream

Place prepared loaf in center third of 12-in. side of Pasta, still on cookie sheet. Wrap the loaf by folding ends up and over; then fold sides over loaf cutting off any overlap more than 3 in. Brush top and sides of loaf with egg and milk beaten together. Bake at 375 degrees until golden brown.

Serves 4.

STEWED TOMATO SALMON

2 lbs. salmon steaks
2 Tbsp. lemon juice
3 Tbsp. butter, melted
Stewed Tomatoes Magnifique (p. 66)

Place salmon on broiling pan. Sprinkle with lemon juice and cover generously with butter. Broil 5 min. Turn. Cover second side with lemon and butter. Continue broiling until done. Top with hot Stewed Tomatoes Magnifique.

Variations:

Try these tomatoes over red snapper.

Prepare shrimp and top with Stewed Tomatoes Magnifique.

Serves 4.

CREAMED TURBOT WITH BACON

2 lbs. turbot, cut into serving pieces
¼ cup butter
4 slices gluten bread
¼ cup butter
½ tsp. salt
¼ tsp. pepper
1 Tbsp. dehydrated parsley flakes
2 cups light cream
½ tsp. thyme
2 Tbsp. lemon juice
⅓ cup onions, chopped fine
8 slices bacon, crisp-fried and crumbled

Cook turbot in ¼ cup butter until tender and white throughout. Combine gluten bread, ¼ cup butter, salt, pepper, parsley flakes, cream, thyme and lemon juice in blender and mix until smooth. Pour into saucepan. Stir in onions and simmer gently until hot but do not allow to boil. Pour sauce over cooked turbot and garnish with bacon bits.

Serves 4.

SWISS-BAKE TURBOT

1 egg
1 Tbsp. milk
1 Tbsp. lemon juice
½ tsp. salt
2 lbs. turbot, cut into serving size pieces
1½ cups Gluten Bread Crumbs (p. 143)
4 Tbsp. butter
1½ cups Swiss Cheese Sauce (p. 59)

Combine egg with milk, lemon juice and salt. Dip turbot first into egg mixture, then coat with Crumbs. Melt butter in pan and add fish. Fry until golden brown on both sides and fish is white inside. Place on serving dishes and top with hot Swiss Cheese Sauce.

Variations:
Substitute Cheese Sauce for Swiss Cheese Sauce.
Use halibut steaks in place of turbot.
Sprinkle chopped parsley over sauce before serving.

Serves 4.

RED SNAPPER WITH DILL SAUCE

2 lbs. red snapper
½ cup onion, diced
1½ Tbsp. butter
2 Tbsp. lemon juice
1 cup dry white wine
¾ tsp. salt
2 cups Dill Sauce (p. 56)

Place fish in pan and cover with onion, butter, lemon juice, wine and salt. Cover and simmer 10 min. Drain and serve with Dill Sauce.

Serves 4.

CRUMB-FRIED SCALLOPS

2 eggs
1 Tbsp. milk
1 Tbsp. lemon juice
2 lbs. scallops
1½ cups Oven-Dried Gluten Bread Crumbs (p. 143)
Equal amounts butter and oil, as needed
1¾ cups Seafood Sauce Marvel (p. 60)

Beat eggs with milk and add lemon juice. Dip scallops in egg mixture, then coat well with Crumbs. Fry in butter and oil until tender and golden brown. Serve with Seafood Sauce Marvel.

Suggestion: Substitute any favorite seafood for scallops.

Serves 4–6.

HAWAIIAN-STYLE KING CRAB

8 Alaska king crab legs, shelled (about 4 oz. ea.)
Salt and pepper, as desired
½ cup light cream
Oven-Dried Gluten Bread Crumbs (p. 143)
Butter, for frying
⅓–½ cup melted butter
1 Tbsp. prepared mustard
Juice from 1 lime
¼ cup parsley, chopped fine

Split each crab leg in half, lengthwise. Sprinkle with salt and pepper. Dip pieces first into cream and then into Crumbs. Sauté breaded legs in butter over medium heat until golden brown on both sides. Mix ⅓–½ cup melted butter with mustard, lime juice and parsley. Pour mixture over crab legs and serve.

Serves 4.

FILLET OF HALIBUT IN DILL

2 lbs. halibut fillets
Water
1 cup onions, diced
1 tsp. coarse ground pepper
1½ tsp. salt
2 Tbsp. lemon juice
½ tsp. dill weed

Place halibut in pan and cover with water. Add onions, pepper, salt, lemon juice and dill weed. Simmer until fish is done, about 20 min. Drain and serve.

Serves 4.

SEAFOOD COMBO DELIGHT

2 cloves garlic, minced
1¼ cups onion, chopped
4 Tbsp. butter
¾ cup dry white wine
1 cup clams, canned, with liquid
1½ cups shrimp
1½ cups oysters
1¼ cups White Cream Sauce, medium (p. 55)
2 generous dashes Tabasco
½ tsp. salt
¼ tsp. pepper
¼ cup chives
Mozzarella or Romano cheese, grated
Gluten Egg Noodles (p. 142)

Add garlic to onion and sauté in butter. Add wine, all fish and liquid from clams, White Cream Sauce, Tabasco, salt and pepper. Stir well and simmer until thoroughly heated. Stir in chives and generous amount of cheese. Serve over Gluten Egg Noodles.

Serves about 6.

TUNA À LA CRÈME

1 cup White Cream Sauce (p. 55)
Dash onion powder
Dash garlic powder
1/8 tsp. cream of tartar
1 can tuna, flaked
Gluten Egg Noodles (p. 142), *or*
2 slices Stretch-Cut Gluten Toast (p. 143)

Combine White Cream Sauce, onion powder, garlic powder and cream of tartar in blender. Pour into a saucepan and add tuna. Cook over low heat until hot but not boiling. Spoon over Gluten Noodles or Toast.

Variation: Substitute flaked salmon for tuna.

Serves 2.

CHEESE-TUNA CASSEROLE

1 cup cottage cheese
1½ cups sour cream
½ cup scallions, chopped
2 cloves garlic, minced
1 Tbsp. Worcestershire sauce
½ tsp. salt
2 cans tuna, drained
Dash Tabasco sauce
Gluten Egg Noodles (p. 142)
½ cup cheddar cheese, grated

Combine cottage cheese, sour cream, scallions, garlic, Worcestershire sauce, salt, tuna and Tabasco. Mix with Noodles, place in well-greased baking pan and top with cheese. Bake at 350 degrees for 30 min.

Serves 4.

STUFFED LOBSTER GRANDEUR

4 lobsters, cleaned and split
¼ cup melted butter
¼ cup lemon juice
3 cups Gluten Bread Crumbs (p. 143)
¾ cup butter
¾ cup light cream
Dry red wine
⅓ cup Parmesan cheese, grated
Paprika, salt and pepper, as desired
Melted butter and lemon wedges

Crack claws of lobsters and brush lobsters with mixture of ¼ cup melted butter and ¼ cup lemon juice. Mix Crumbs, ¾ cup butter and cream. Use wine to moisten mixture. Stuff lobster cavities; then sprinkle with cheese and paprika. Place in lined pan and broil at least 6 inches from heat until flesh turns opaque-white and shell turns red. Season with salt and pepper; serve with melted butter and lemon wedges.

Serves 4.

CHICKEN HONOLULU STYLE

6–8 chicken parts
Salt, as desired
Dash white pepper
1 egg
⅓ cup unsweetened orange juice concentrate
Sugar substitute equivalent to 1 tsp. sugar
¾ cup Gluten Bread Crumbs (p. 143)
⅔ cup fresh coconut, shredded
½ cup butter, melted

Season chicken with salt and pepper. Combine egg, orange juice and sugar substitute. Combine Crumbs, coconut and 2½ Tbsp. butter. Dip chicken pieces into egg mixture, then coat evenly in Crumb mixture. Place chicken in buttered dish and bake at 350 degrees for 45 min. Pour remaining butter over chicken and bake for an additional 15 min.

Serves 4–6.

CHICKEN WITH GINGER SAUCE

2½ cups chicken, cooked and diced
1¾ cups Ginger Sauce (p. 53)
Gluten Egg Noodles (p. 142)

Heat chicken pieces in Ginger Sauce. Pour over Noodles and serve.

Variation: Replace chicken with turkey.

Serves 2–4.

SOY-GLAZED CHICKEN

½ cup lemon juice
3 Tbsp. soy sauce
¾ tsp. oregano
¼ tsp. salt
Dash pepper
Dash garlic powder
Dash onion powder
1 cup oil
1 broiler-fryer chicken, quartered (approx. 3 lbs.)

Mix all ingredients. Marinate chicken 5 to 6 hrs. Bring wing tips onto cut side or back. Place chicken in pan for broiling. Broil 5–6 in. from heat source for 20 min. Turn skin side up and broil an additional 10 min. or until chicken is done. Brush often during broiling with soy glaze.

Serves 3–4.

BLEU CHEESE CHICKEN

- ¾ cup bleu cheese
- 1 cup cold water
- ½ cup non-fat dry milk
- 2 cups small curd cottage cheese
- Juice from 1 small lemon (about 2 Tbsp.)
- ¼–⅓ tsp. onion powder
- ¼ tsp. salt
- 1 (3½ lb.) chicken, cut into pieces
- Oil and butter

Mix ½ cup bleu cheese, water, dry milk, cottage cheese, lemon juice, onion powder and salt in blender until smooth. Stir in remaining ¼ cup bleu cheese, crumbled. Rinse chicken pieces, drain and pat dry. Marinate in half of the cheese mixture 6 hrs. or overnight. Put small amount of oil in frying pan and brown chicken lightly on all sides. Remove to hot generously buttered baking pan. Spoon desired amount of cheese mixture over top. Cover and bake at 350 degrees for 1 hr. or until chicken is tender. (If there is any excess cheese mixture, store it to be used later as salad dressing.)

Variations: Replace bleu cheese mixture with any favorite allowed salad dressing.

Serves 4.

TURKEY PIE

- 1½ cups White Cream Sauce (p. 55)
- ¼ tsp. thyme
- ½ cup celery, diced
- Turkey, cooked and diced, to fill pie pan as desired
- Gluten Pasta, baked in pie pan until set (p. 142)
- Green pepper strips

Mix White Cream Sauce with thyme. Add celery and turkey. Heat gently. Pour into pan containing partially baked Pasta. Top with green pepper strips and put into 350 degree oven until Pasta has completed baking and turkey is hot. Serve immediately.

Serves 2–4.

CURRIED TURKEY CASSEROLE

2 cups White Cream Sauce (p. 55)
¼ tsp. curry powder
¼ tsp. ginger
4 cups turkey, cooked and cut into bite-size pieces
Gluten Egg Noodles (p. 142)

To White Cream Sauce, add curry powder and ginger. Stir in turkey pieces. Heat slowly, then spoon over warm Noodles.

Serves 2–4.

TURKEY WITH TOMATO-CHEESE SAUCE

Turkey, cooked and cut into bite-size pieces
1 cup Tomato-Cheese Sauce (p. 58)
Gluten Egg Noodles (p. 142)
Water, to thin sauce during cooking

Stir turkey pieces into sauce and heat slowly until turkey is hot. Serve over noodles.

Variation: Try diced chicken with Tomato-Cheese Sauce.

Serves 2–4.

CHEESE BLINTZES

Crepes:
2 slices gluten bread
4 eggs
1 tsp. butter, melted
¼ tsp. salt
½ cup milk

Process all ingredients in blender until smooth. Pour small amount of batter into center of buttered, heated pan of desired size, rotating the pan so that the batter spreads evenly. Fry over medium heat until edges are lightly browned and top is beginning to set and bubble slightly. Place on wax paper by turning pan upside down and tapping lightly, if necessary, to loosen crepe. May be stacked between pieces of wax paper until needed.

Filling:
1 lb. hoop cheese (or ricotta)
½ tsp. lemon juice
Sugar substitute equivalent to 1½ tsp. sugar
¾ tsp. vanilla extract
2 eggs
Generous 2 Tbsp. butter, softened

Mix all ingredients well. Spoon 2 Tbsp. of filling into center of each crepe. Wrap by folding bottom side up, side over and top down. Fry 3 min. on each side in buttered pan.

Suggestion: Serve with sour cream or sugarless applesauce. These are a rare treat!

Makes approximately 10 blintzes.

TUNA MELT CREPES

Crepes (see Cheese Blintzes, above)
10 Swiss cheese slices
2 cans tuna, flaked, with mayonnaise, *or*
Favorite tuna salad

Prepare Crepes. Cut 1 slice cheese in half lengthwise. Place half in center of crepe. Spoon 2 Tbsp. tuna mixture over cheese and top with other half cheese slice. Fold and fry as for Cheese Blintzes.

Makes 10.

Desserts and Drinks

CINNAMON-APPLE TOPPING

1 med. apple
Water
1½ tsp. Cinnamon Sprinkle (p. 115)

Peel apple and dice into very small pieces. Place pieces in small saucepan and cover with water. Add Cinnamon Sprinkle and stir. Cover and cook over medium heat until soft, about 10 min.

Makes ½ cup.

BUTTERSCOTCH SAUCE

2 envelopes butterscotch diet pudding
⅔–¾ cup water
Sugar substitute equivalent to ¼ cup sugar
2 tsp. butter

Combine pudding with water and sugar substitute. Bring to a full, rolling boil. Remove from heat and stir in butter. Serve warm over dessert cakes, pies and frosts.

Makes about 1 cup.

VANILLA SAUCE

Follow recipe for Butterscotch Sauce substituting vanilla pudding for butterscotch.

Variations: Add extract of your choice to vanilla flavor pudding for great variety of dessert sauces.

CHOCOLATE SAUCE

Follow recipe for Butterscotch Sauce substituting chocolate pudding for butterscotch.

ORANGE SAUCE

- 2 egg yolks
- 4 tsp. orange juice
- 2 tsp. powdered non-fat milk
- Sugar substitute equivalent to 3 tsp. sugar
- 4 Tbsp. melted butter

Combine all ingredients except butter in blender and process at low speed until thoroughly mixed. With blender running, pour butter steadily into mixture. Chill until thick. Serve over pancakes, waffles, desserts.

Makes ¼ cup.

ORANGE SAUCE SUPREME

- 2 med. oranges
- ¼ cup vodka
- Sugar substitute equivalent to ½ cup sugar
- 1 Tbsp. lemon juice
- ¼ cup water
- 2 egg yolks

Remove peel from oranges and grate. Soak grated rind in vodka for about 45 min. Squeeze oranges, adding more juice if necessary, to make 1 cup juice. Combine juice with sugar substitute, lemon juice, water and rind with vodka. Pour into double boiler over hot water, stir in egg yolks. Heat, stirring constantly, until mixture thickens. Serve over pancakes, crepes, fruit or dessert pastries.

Makes 1½ cups.

PASTRY CRUST

2 slices gluten bread
2 eggs
¼ cup light cream
¼ cup milk
Sugar substitute equivalent to 3 tsp. sugar
1 tsp. vanilla flavoring

Combine all ingredients in blender until smooth. Follow directions for Gluten Pasta (p. 142) using all but ½ cup of this batter on a cookie sheet.

Makes 1 10-in. x 15-in. crust.

IMPERIAL CHEESE CAKE

1½ cups Oven-Dried Gluten Bread Crumbs (p. 143)
Liquid sugar substitute equivalent to ½ cup sugar
2 tsp. vanilla extract
¼ cup cold water
2 (8 oz.) pkgs. cream cheese, softened
5 egg yolks
¼ tsp. salt
2 tsp. vanilla extract
1½ tsp. lemon rind, grated
2 Tbsp. lemon juice
1 cup sour cream
5 egg whites
½ cup Cream Frosting (p. 115)

Combine Crumbs, sugar substitute, 1 tsp. vanilla and water. Press ¾ of the mixture into 9-in. spring form pan. Bake at 325 degrees for 5 min. Combine all remaining ingredients except egg whites and frosting. Beat until well blended. Beat egg whites until stiff and fold into cheese mixture. Turn into spring form pan. Bake at 325 degrees until set, about 1 hr.

Spread with Cream Frosting and return to oven for 5 min. or until frosting is firm. Cool 1½ hrs. Remove collar from pan and top with remaining ¼ of crumb mixture.

Serves 8.

PIE SHELL DELUXE

1 egg
Sugar substitute equivalent to 2 tsp. sugar
1 tsp. vanilla flavoring
2 Tbsp. milk
1 slice gluten bread
2 Tbsp. light cream

Combine all ingredients in blender until smooth. Pre-heat oven at 425 degrees for 15 min. Place generously greased or non-stick 8-in. pie pan in oven for 3 min. Remove pan and pour in pastry mixture, rotating pan to allow mixture to set evenly on bottom and around sides. Return pan to oven and bake 8 min. Cool.

Makes 1 8-in. shell.

CUSTARD SAUCE

1½ cups milk
Scant dash salt
Sugar substitute equivalent to 2 Tbsp. sugar
3 egg yolks, slightly beaten
1 tsp. vanilla

Scald milk, add salt and sugar substitute. Add egg yolks. Cook in top of double boiler, stirring constantly, until thickened. Cool and stir in vanilla.

Suggestion: Spoon over allowed fruits.

Variations: Add almond or coconut extract and serve over strawberries.

Makes 1½ cups.

APPLE TURNOVERS

Pastry Crust (p. 182)
Cinnamon-Apple Topping (p. 180)
2 tsp. Cinnamon Sprinkle (p. 115)
1 egg white
Butter

Cut Pastry Crust into 6 squares with sharp knife or pizza cutter. Brush both sides of each square well with egg white. Spoon Cinnamon-Apple Topping onto one triangle of each square, leaving room around edges to seal. Fold into triangles, use additional egg white between layers around edges if necessary, and press firmly to seal. Sprinkle tops with Cinnamon Sprinkle. Place on buttered cookie sheet and bake at 450 degrees for 10 min. or until edges are brown and turnover is stiff. Cool.

Variation for Strict Diet: Use Strawberry Jam.

Makes 6.

APPLE CUSTARD PUDDING

1 slice gluten bread, quartered
1 egg
¼–⅓ tsp. cinnamon
Sugar substitute equivalent to 1¼ tsp. sugar
¼ tsp. vanilla extract
½ cup milk
1 med. apple, peeled and sliced thin

Place bread in small baking dish. Beat egg with cinnamon, sugar substitute, vanilla and milk. Pour half of mixture over bread, layer in apple and add remaining half of mixture over top. Bake at 350 degrees for 50 min. or until custard sets and apples are soft.

Serves 1 or 2.

CHOCOLATE-BRANDY PUDDING

1 envelope chocolate diet pudding
½ tsp. imitation brandy flavoring
Whipped cream
Crushed nuts

Follow package directions for preparing pudding. Add brandy flavoring near end of cooking time. When cooled, top with whipped cream and crushed nuts of your choice.

Serves 4.

VANILLA-BUTTERSCOTCH PUDDING

1 envelope butterscotch diet pudding
¾ tsp. vanilla flavoring
Whipped cream

Follow package directions for pudding. Add vanilla flavoring after pudding is dissolved and cook until it comes to a boil. Refrigerate until set. Top with whipped cream.

Serves 4.

CHOCOLATE-ALMOND PUDDING

1 envelope chocolate diet pudding
2 cups milk
½ tsp. almond extract
Whipping cream
Slivered almonds

Dissolve pudding in milk and add extract. Cook, stirring constantly, over medium heat until mixture comes to a boil. Refrigerate until firm. Whip cream; top pudding with it and add slivered almonds.

Serves 4.

VANILLA-SPICE FLUFF

1 envelope vanilla diet pudding
2 cups milk
Sugar substitute equivalent to 2 tsp. sugar
1 egg white
¼ tsp. allspice
Sugar substitute equivalent to 1 tsp. sugar

Mix pudding, milk and equivalent of 2 tsp. sugar in saucepan. Cook over medium heat, stirring until mixture comes to a boil. Beat egg white, allspice and equivalent of 1 tsp. sugar until foamy. Slowly stir in cooked pudding mixture. Sprinkle lightly with nutmeg and chill.

Serves 4.

BUTTERSCOTCH-RUM PUDDING

1 envelope butterscotch diet pudding
Just less than ½ tsp. imitation rum flavoring

Cook pudding according to package directions, adding rum flavoring when pudding is dissolved. Refrigerate.

Serves 4.

COCONUT PUDDING

1 envelope vanilla diet pudding
2 cups milk
Sugar substitute equivalent to 1 tsp. sugar
¼ tsp. lemon extract
⅛ tsp. imitation coconut flavoring *or*
½ cup coconut, shredded

Dissolve pudding in milk and add other ingredients. Stir over medium heat until mixture comes to a boil. (Fold in shredded coconut, if using it.) Chill.

Serves 4.

CHERRY PUDDING

1 envelope vanilla diet pudding
2 cups milk
¼ tsp. imitation cherry flavoring
3 or 4 drops red food coloring

Dissolve pudding in milk and add remaining ingredients. Stir over medium heat until mixture comes to a boil. Pour into dessert cups and refrigerate until firm.

Serves 4.

BANANA-RUM PUDDING

1 envelope vanilla diet pudding
2 cups milk
¼ tsp. banana flavoring
⅛–¼ tsp. imitation rum flavoring

Dissolve pudding in milk and add remaining ingredients. Cook, stirring constantly, over medium heat until mixture comes to a boil. Refrigerate in dessert cups.

Serves 4.

PEACH PUDDING

1 (16 oz.) can diet peach slices
1 envelope vanilla diet pudding
1½ cups milk
Whipped cream

Drain peaches, reserving liquid. Combine pudding and milk slowly over medium heat. Stir in liquid from peaches. Bring to a boil, stirring constantly. Chill, fold in peaches and top pudding with whipped cream.

Variation: Any canned diet fruit may be substituted for peaches.

Serves 4–6.

PUDDING WITH A TANG

1 envelope vanilla diet pudding
¾ cup milk
1¼ cups lemon-lime diet soda

Prepare pudding according to package directions, using milk and soda. Stir before serving.

Variations:

Chocolate pudding with diet ginger ale.
Vanilla pudding with grape or orange diet soda.
Butterscotch pudding with diet ginger ale.
Vanilla pudding with grapefruit diet soda.

Serves 4.

BLUEBERRY PUDDING

1 envelope vanilla diet pudding
2 cups milk
¼ cup blueberries, slightly mashed
Sugar substitute equivalent to 2½ tsp. sugar
2 drops imitation brandy
2 drops red food coloring
Chopped nuts

Empty pudding into saucepan and slowly add milk as you stir. Cook over medium heat until pudding dissolves. Add blueberries, sugar substitute, imitation brandy, and food coloring. Continue to cook, stirring constantly, until mixture just comes to a boil. Remove from heat and pour into dessert dishes. Chill. Serve with chopped nuts sprinkled over top.

Serves 4.

SPEEDY MOCK CUSTARD

3 cups milk
1 envelope vanilla diet pudding
¼–½ tsp. imitation flavoring

Gradually stir milk into pudding in saucepan. Add flavoring and continue stirring over medium heat until mixture comes to a boil. Empty into bowl and chill, stirring occasionally.

Variations:

Use vanilla diet pudding and milk omitting flavoring.

Add imitation almond extract to whipping cream and top mock custard when chilled.

Omit flavoring and top with whipped cream sprinkled with nutmeg.

Serves 6.

APRICOT MERINGUE

- 12 egg whites
- Sugar substitute equivalent to 2½ cups sugar
- 2 tsp. vanilla
- 1 tsp. lemon juice
- 2 tsp. cream of tartar
- Gluten flour
- 1 pt. heavy cream
- ½ (1 lb.) can apricots, seeds removed, chopped fine

Beat egg whites for 1 min. Continue beating while adding sugar substitute. Add vanilla, lemon juice and cream of tartar. Beat until mixture begins to dry. Lightly flour bundt pan with gluten flour. Spoon in meringue and place bundt pan in a pan of hot water. Bake at 275 degrees for about 3½ hrs. Turn onto plate, cool and refrigerate until thoroughly chilled. Whip cream and fold in apricot bits. Frost top and sides of meringue with cream mixture.

Variations:

Serve with Brandy Sauce.

Serve with Rum Sauce.

Replace apricots with blueberries, peaches or strawberries.

Serves 10.

CHEESE ROLL DELIGHT

Pastry Crust (p. 182)
1 egg white
8 oz. sharp cheddar cheese, sliced thin
Butter

Thoroughly brush Pastry Crust on both sides with egg white. Cut into 12 triangles. Cut cheese slices into slightly smaller triangles. Place one piece of cheese on each piece of crust. Roll diagonally and press to seal, using additional egg white if necessary. Bake on buttered cookie sheet at 450 degrees until cheese melts and crust is crisp, about 7 min.

Suggestion: Serve with fruit for dessert.

Variations:

These variations make delicious hors d'oeuvres.

Cut crust into squares, place diced tomatoes over cheese and seal as for a turnover.

Sprinkle cheese with celery seeds before rolling.

Cut crust into squares and use cooked bacon bits over cheese.

Makes 12.

APPLE-PECAN TURNOVERS

Cinnamon-Apple Topping (p. 180)
1 egg white
Pastry Crust (p. 182)
⅓–½ cup pecans, chopped fine
1½ tsp. Cinnamon Sprinkle (p. 115)

Follow directions for Apple Turnovers (p. 184), adding pecans over Cinnamon-Apple Topping.

Variations:

Substitute walnuts for pecans.

Use ¼ cup Brazil nuts and ¼ cup cashews instead of pecans.

Makes 6.

HOT FRUIT COMBO

1 (1 lb.) can plums
1 (1 lb.) can apricots
1 (1 lb.) can pears
Liquid from combined fruits, as needed
Whipped cream
Nutmeg

Combine plums, apricots, pears and liquid in saucepan. Heat slowly until piping hot. Serve combination of fruit with liquid spooned over top. Garnish with whipped cream and sprinkle with nutmeg.

Suggestions: This dish is a unique addition to a cold seafood salad meal. Hot fruit makes an inviting dessert. It may be topped with whipped cream flavored with extracts or sprinkled with shredded coconut.

Serves about 10.

CINNAMON NUT ROLLS

Pastry Crust (p. 182)
1 egg white
¼ cup pecans, chopped
1½ Tbsp. almonds, chopped
1½ Tbsp. cashews, chopped
1 Tbsp. Cinnamon Sprinkle (p. 115)
Butter

Cut Pastry Crust into 6 rectangles. Thoroughly brush each with egg white on both sides. Mix nuts. Spread 1 Tbsp. nut mixture over each rectangle, leaving edges free. Spread Cinnamon Sprinkle (¼ tsp. each) over nuts. Begin at one corner of each rectangle and roll diagonally. Secure with egg white if necessary; press to seal. Top each roll with ⅛ tsp. Cinnamon Sprinkle. Place on buttered cookie sheet and bake at 450 degrees for 6–8 min.

Makes 6.

GRILLED APPLE COBBLER

Butter
1 slice gluten bread, crust removed
Cinnamon-Apple Topping (p. 180)

Melt butter in frying pan until it bubbles. Drop bread onto hot pan and turn immediately, coating first side with butter. Flatten with spatula as it browns. Turn and repeat. Remove to plate and top with hot Cinnamon-Apple Topping.

Serves 1.

APRICOTS FLAMBÉ

2 (1 lb.) cans apricot halves
¼ cup butter, melted
Sugar substitute equivalent to 2 tsp. sugar
¼ cup brandy

Drain apricots and place in shallow pan for broiling. Drizzle with butter and sprinkle with sugar substitute. Broil until apricots are lightly browned. Remove to warm chafing dish. Pour brandy over apricots and flame.

Variations:
Substitute peaches or pears for apricots.
Top with whipped cream.

Serves 6.

CREAM CHEESE FINGER PASTRIES

Pastry Crust (p. 182)
1 egg white
3 oz. whipped cream cheese
⅓–½ cup walnuts, chopped
Butter

Cut baked Pastry Crust into 6 squares. Generously brush each on both sides with egg white. Spread thin layer of cheese on each and top with 1 Tbsp. walnuts, keeping filling to within ¼ in. of edges. Roll diagonally and press lightly to secure. Place pastries on buttered cookie sheet and bake at 450 degrees until cheese is hot and crust is firm and golden.

Makes 6.

APPLE MACAROONS

- 1½ cups apples, peeled, cored and grated
- Brown sugar substitute equivalent to ¼ cup sugar
- 1 tsp. cinnamon
- 1 tsp. coconut extract
- 2⅔ cups powdered non-fat milk
- ⅓ cup coconut, grated

Combine all ingredients, mixing well, and spoon immediately onto non-stick cookie sheet. Bake at 350 degrees until lightly browned.

Variations:

Use maple extract and pecans.
Substitute almond extract and chopped mixed nuts.
Use fruit extracts with coconut or nut mixtures.

Makes about 4 dozen cookies.

COCONUT MOCHA

- 2 envelopes vanilla diet pudding
- ⅔ tsp. vanilla extract
- ⅔ tsp. instant decaffeinated coffee
- ½ tsp. coconut extract
- Shredded coconut

Prepare pudding according to package instructions. Stir in vanilla and divide mixture in half. Add coffee to first half and coconut extract to remaining half. Layer into parfait glasses and top with shredded coconut.

Serves 8.

MACADAMIA RUM ROLLS

¼ cup light cream
¼ cup milk
2 eggs
2 slices gluten bread
Sugar substitute equivalent to 4 tsp. sugar
1 tsp. rum flavoring
1 egg white
½ cup macadamia nuts, chopped
Butter

Combine cream, milk, eggs, bread, sugar substitute and rum flavoring in blender. Process until smooth. Bake as for Gluten Pasta. Cut baked crust into 6 rectangles. Brush both sides of each with egg white. Spoon about 1 Tbsp. nuts onto each and spread to within ¼ in. of edges. Roll diagonally, from corner to corner, and press to seal. Place on buttered cookie sheet and bake at 450 degrees for 6–8 min. until lightly browned and stiff.

Makes 6.

ORANGE SHERBET

½ cup milk
3 Tbsp. concentrated frozen orange juice
Sugar substitute, to taste

Place all ingredients in blender and process until smooth. Freeze for 1 hr. only. (If freezing sherbet longer, remove from freezer 10 min. before serving.)

Variations for Strict Diet:

Add imitation flavorings to light cream and freeze until desired consistency is achieved.

Add extracts to sugarless diet sodas. Freeze as above.

Serves 1.

PINEAPPLE-COCONUT COOKIES

2 egg whites, at room temperature
1 tsp. coconut extract
1¼ tsp. vanilla extract
½ cup Gluten Bread Crumbs (p. 143)
2½ tsp. pineapple extract

Beat egg whites until soft peaks form. Beat in coconut and vanilla extracts until stiff. Combine Crumbs with pineapple extract and mix well. Add a few drops of water if all crumbs are not moistened. Fold whites into Crumbs. Form cookies and place on non-stick or well-greased cookie sheet. Bake at 300 degrees for 15 min. Remove and cool.

Suggestion: Be creative about changing extracts.

Makes about 1 dozen.

CREPES WITH CHOCOLATE SAUCE

French Pancakes (p. 146)
2 envelopes chocolate diet pudding
⅔–¾ cup water
Sugar substitute equivalent to ¼ cup sugar
2 tsp. butter

Prepare French Pancakes and remove to warm oven. Mix pudding with water and sugar substitute. Bring to a full bubbling boil. Remove from heat and stir in butter. Serve warm over French Pancakes.

Suggestion: This sauce may be used over a variety of desserts and it is very good cold.

Variations: Replace chocolate diet pudding with butterscotch or vanilla for marvelous dessert sauces. They may be flavored with a variety of imitation flavorings. (See Puddings.)

Serves 6.

BANANA CREAM PIE

2 envelopes vanilla diet pudding
3½ cups milk
Sugar substitute equivalent to 1 Tbsp. sugar
¾ tsp. imitation banana flavoring
1 Pie Shell Deluxe (p. 183)
Whipped cream, as desired, for topping

Empty pudding into saucepan and slowly add milk. Stir over medium heat just until pudding is dissolved. Add sugar substitute and banana flavoring. Continue cooking until mixture begins to boil. Stir 2 times during 5 min. cooling period. Pour into prepared Pie Shell Deluxe (cooled) and refrigerate at least 2 hrs. Top with whipped cream just before serving.

Makes 1 8-in. pie.

NO-BAKE PEANUT BUTTER COOKIES

½ cup chunky peanut butter
½ cup coconut, shredded
½ cup powdered non-fat milk
Brown sugar substitute equivalent to 1 Tbsp. sugar
1 Tbsp. orange rind, grated
1 Tbsp. orange juice
Powdered non-fat milk, if desired for coating

In mixing bowl, combine peanut butter with coconut. Add remaining ingredients, taking care to mix thoroughly. Form crumbly mixture into balls and roll in powdered milk if desired. Chill in refrigerator or freeze.

Variation: Mix peanut butter, milk and orange juice. Roll mixture flat between two pieces of wax paper; score and freeze.

Makes 18–20.

MOCK ORANGE JULIUS

- 4 ice cubes
- 1 medium orange, peeled and cut
- ½ cup water
- 1 tsp. vanilla extract
- Sugar substitute equivalent to 2 tsp. sugar

Combine all ingredients in blender and process until foamy.

Makes 1½ cups.

Index